Vitamins and "Health" Foods: The Great American Hustle

Vitamins and "Health" Foods:

The Great American Hustle

VICTOR HERBERT, M.D., J.D.
Professor of Medicine
State University of New York
Downstate Medical Center;
Chief, Hematology and Nutrition Laboratory
Bronx VA Medical Center

and

STEPHEN BARRETT, M.D.
Chairman, Board of Directors
Lehigh Valley Committee Against Health Fraud, Inc.

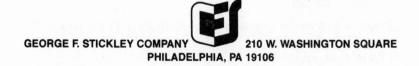

GEORGE F. STICKLEY COMPANY   210 W. WASHINGTON SQUARE
PHILADELPHIA, PA 19106

Vitamins and "Health" Foods:

The Great American Hustle is a special publication of the Lehigh Valley Committee Against Health Fraud, Inc., an independent organization which was formed in 1969 to combat deception in the field of health. The purposes of the Committee are:

1. To investigate false, deceptive or exaggerated health claims.
2. To conduct a vigorous campaign of public education.
3. To assist appropriate government and consumer-oriented agencies.
4. To bring problems to the attention of lawmakers.

The Lehigh Valley Committee Against Health Fraud is a member organization of the Consumer Federation of America. Since 1970, the Committee has been chartered under the laws of the Commonwealth of Pennsylvania as a not-for-profit corporation. Inquiries about Committee activities may be addressed to P.O. Box 1602, Allentown, PA 18105.

Third Printing May 1982.
Copyright © 1981, Lehigh Valley Committee Against
Health Fraud, Inc.
ISBN 0-89313-054-0   LCC # 81-83596

Manufactured in the United States of America; Published by the George F. Stickley Company, 210 W. Washington Square, Philadelphia, PA. 19106.

Contents

About the Authors

Victor Herbert, M.D., J.D., is Chief of the Hematology and Nutrition Laboratory, Bronx VA Medical Center and Professor of Medicine at State University of New York Downstate Medical Center. He is board-certified in internal medicine and nutrition, has taught full-time at five major medical schools, and has been a visiting professor at most other medical schools in the United States and Canada. A member of many scientific societies, he has published over 500 articles and is the author of *Nutrition Cultism: Facts and Fictions*. He received the 1972 McCollum Award of the American Society of Clinical Nutrition and the 1978 Middleton Award of the Veterans Administration in recognition of his outstanding research in nutrition. He has testified several times before Congress on health and nutrition subjects and has served as a medicolegal expert for the U.S. government and several state governments. He is a member of the Food and Nutrition Board of the National Academy of Sciences and of its Recommended Dietary Allowances (RDA) Committee. He is a member of the Joint Subcommittee on Human Nutrition Research of the Executive Office of the President, and was for five years Chairman of the Committee on Life Sciences of the American Bar Association. Past-President of the American Society for Clinical Nutrition, he is the only person in the world listed in both *World Who's Who in Science* and *Who's Who in American Law*. He is also listed in *Science Citation Index* as one of the scientists most cited by other scientists throughout the world.

Stephen Barrett, M.D., a practicing psychiatrist and lecturer on consumer health, is the nation's most vigorous opponent of health quackery. Since 1970, he has been Board Chairman of the Lehigh Valley Committee Against Health Fraud, Inc., a member organization of Consumer Federation of America. An expert in medical communications, he serves as medical consultant to WFMZ-TV, Allentown, Pa., and as Consumer Health Editor of *Nautilus Magazine.* He is editor of *The Health Robbers* (a comprehensive expose of quackery), co-editor of *The Tooth Robbers: A Pro-Fluoridation Handbook,* and co-author of the college textbook *Consumer Health—A Guide to Intelligent Decisions,* all published in 1980. He has been a member of the Committee on Quackery of the Pennsylvania Medical Society and the Committee on Health Fraud of the Pennsylvania Health Council. He is a scientific advisor to the American Council on Science and Health and a scientific consultant to the Committee for Scientific Investigation of Claims of the Paranormal (CSICOP).

Foreword

Do you get angry when someone tries to hustle you? Would it bother you if someone promised you something and took your money, but gave you nothing in return? Do you think you have ever been hustled without realizing it?

What goes through your mind when you see an ad which suggests that a pill can help you lose weight permanently without dieting or exercising? If it doesn't strike you as phony, you don't know the facts. There is no such pill.

How about a magazine article which claims that a single drug can make you a better athlete, help you live longer, cure heart disease, diabetes, cancer, gallbladder pain and a host of other ailments? If you think such a drug exists, you had better read this book.

Do you take vitamin pills? Has it occurred to you to question whether you really need them? You should. Most of the more than 70 million Americans who take them are merely nourishing their toilets and making vitamin manufacturers rich.

But the issue is not simply one of wasted money. Each decision you make about your health must be based upon an underlying judgment about whom to trust for advice. *If you cannot tell the difference between an expert and a hustler, you are likely to be misled.*

One of the factors that makes America great is our freedom of speech. To maintain this freedom, we must also run a risk. False prophets can get up on pedestals and tell you almost anything they please.

Such prophets abound in the field of nutrition. One reason they succeed is that too many people who know better are afraid to become involved in controversy.

The people who wrote this book *are* involved. Dr. Herbert has done more to attack nutrition frauds than any other person in America. He has testified before legislatures and courts. He spent his own money seeking justice. He is one of the most knowledgeable and respected nutrition experts in the country—one to whom other experts turn frequently for advice.

Dr. Barrett has investigated and written about quackery in more and different fields than any other living American. He has written about health, medical care, drugs, nutrition, the environment and the workplace.

This is one book you should not ignore. It is one of the most amazing investigative reports in the history of journalism. It is likely to save you money. It might even save your life!

GABE MIRKIN, M.D.

Dr. Mirkin, a practicing physician who specializes in allergy, immunology, dermatology and sportsmedicine, is Assistant Professor of Sportsmedicine at the University of Maryland. An expert on fitness and nutrition, he is co-author of *The Sportsmedicine Book* and writes regularly for the New York Times Syndicate and several sports magazines. He is also Daily Fitness Broadcaster for the CBS Radio Network.

Introduction

One of the lessons of Watergate is that questionable operations involving large sums of money are likely to create a "paper trail" of incriminating evidence. The "health" food industry—which has been selling its bill of goods for many years—is no exception.

This book is based upon 10 years of investigation. Like the Watergate story, it was inspired by a few "defectors" who provided documents that were never intended for public view. Our survey of trade publications, combined with material in our files and a modest amount of undercover investigation, then brought the whole seamy picture into focus.

The sale of unnecessary and sometimes dangerous food supplements is a multibillion dollar industry. This book endeavors to answer four questions:

How is the "health" food industry organized?
How do its salespeople learn their trade?
How many people are involved?
Most important, *how do they get away with what they are doing?*

Chapter 1

The Truth About Nutrition

Most people who take vitamins don't need them. Could you be one of these people? Are you afraid there is not enough nourishment in the food you buy?

Do you think that vitamin pills can give you extra energy? That extra vitamins should be taken in times of stress? That vitamin C can prevent colds? Or that large doses of other nutrients can prevent or cure many other ailments?

Are you afraid that there are "too many chemicals" in our food? Do you think that foods labeled "natural" or "organic" are safer or more nutritious?

If you have any of these fears or beliefs, you have plenty of company. But you have been misled!

America is in the midst of a vitamin craze. Health hustlers who spread false ideas have developed a huge public following. But nutrition is not a religion. It is a science—human biochemistry. What a nutrient can or cannot do in the body is determined by its specific chemical structure and the specific biochemical reactions in which that structure can become involved.

How can you tell what to believe? The answer to this question has two parts. First, you should know what is meant by "scientific truth." Then you must determine who is telling the truth.

How Do We Know What We "Know"?

How are medical facts determined? Mankind has always been curious about disease and what causes it. The more we understand, of course, the better we can control illness. Down through the centuries, countless people have shared their observations and ideas. Thousands of speculations have been offered to explain what people saw. During the past century, however, ideas have developed which seem to make more sense than others before them. Armed with these ideas, man has been able to cure many diseases in an almost miraculous fashion. As part of this process of scientific development, good methods have been developed to test whether proposed theories are correct. The sum of these meth-

1

ods is known as the "experimental" or "scientific" method. This method is used to answer questions like: "If two things happen, one after the other, are they related?" For example, suppose you take a pill when you have a headache and the headache goes away one hour later. How can we tell whether the pill relieved you or whether the headache would have gone away by itself anyway? Throughout the world, hundreds of thousands of scientists are working continuously to determine the boundaries of scientific thought.

As mountains of information are collected, how can we tell which evidence is valid? "Valid" means honestly collected and properly interpreted—using good techniques of statistical analysis. One hallmark of a good experiment is that others can repeat it and get the same results.

This brings us to the question of who can best interpret experimental findings. Scientists are judging each other all the time. People with equal or superior training look for loopholes in each others' experimental techniques and design other experiments to test conclusions. Skilled reviewers also gather in groups whose levels of ability far exceed that of the average scientist. Such experts are not likely to be misled by poorly designed experiments. Among the reviewers are editors and editorial boards of scientific journals who require scientists to fully explain how they did their experiments and how they validated their conclusions. These reviewers carefully screen out invalid findings and publish significant ones in scientific journals. (Most responsible journals that cover nutrition topics are listed in the *Index Medicus* of the National Library of Medicine.) Gradually a shared set of beliefs is developed which is felt to be scientifically accurate. When we speak of the "scientific community," we refer to this overall process of determining what is scientific truth and what is not. In the field of nutrition, the most respected scientific body is the Food and Nutrition Board of the National Research Council, National Academy of Sciences.

Quacks, of course, operate outside of the scientific community. They do not use the scientific method to evaluate what they see. In fact, they seldom bother to experiment at all. When scientists point out that they are wrong, quacks try to cover up their inadequacies by pointing out that the scientific community has made mistakes in the past. This, of course, is true, but irrelevant. In recent years, the chances of major error by the scientific community have decreased greatly. So if you find someone referred to as a "scientist ahead of his time," he is probably a quack. Quacks may boast of "thousands of cases" in their files. But they won't tell you that none of these cases separates cause and effect from coincidence or misdiagnosis.

Basic Principles

Many people think that to achieve good health they must know what each nutrient does in the body. This is absolutely untrue! You don't need to know the biochemical properties of specific nutrients any more than you must know how the parts of a car work in order to be a good driver. Running the human machine, from a nutritional point of view, is quite simple. You need to recognize only four basic facts:

1. All the nutrients you need can be obtained by eating a balanced *variety* of foods.
2. Body weight is a matter of *arithmetic*. If you eat more calories than you need, you will gain weight. To lose weight, you must burn off more calories than you take in.
3. The basic principle of healthy eating is *moderation* in all things.
4. No proposed remedy should be considered safe or effective until *proved* to be safe or effective.

Recommended Dietary Allowances

In 1943, the Food and Nutrition Board began publishing nutrient guidelines which have been revised at approximately 5-year intervals as new scientific data have become available. Known as the "Recommended Dietary Allowances (RDAs)," they are defined as "the levels of intake of essential nutrients considered, in the judgment of the Committee on Dietary Allowances of the Food and Nutrition Board on the basis of available scientific knowledge, to be adequate to meet the known nutritional needs of practically all healthy persons." The committee which developed the most recently published (1980) RDAs was composed of nine recognized nutrition experts, one each from Massachusetts Institute of Technology, Michigan State University, the National Institutes of Health, the U.S. Department of Agriculture, the Letterman Army Institute of Research, and the Universities of California, Iowa, Michigan and Alabama.

RDAs should not be confused with "requirements." They are deliberately set higher than most people need. The RDA for each vitamin and mineral is usually set by noting the entire range of normal human needs, selecting the number at the high end of that range, and adding a "safety factor" to allow for "reserve" body stores without risking toxicity from overdosage. For example, the range of normal adult need for vitamin C is 5-10 mg per day. In setting the RDA at 60 mg, a 50 mg "safety factor" is added so that the body will store 1,500 mg of vitamin C, enough to last five months if you ate no vitamin C at all.

Quacks often charge that the RDAs are set by a group which has a "conflict of interest" to work to benefit the food industry. If you ever hear this, don't believe it. There is not one representative of industry on this committee. Its work is supported by the National Institutes of Health, but members themselves serve without pay. Meeting at regular intervals, the committee sets its values after thorough study of the best evidence that scientists all over the world have developed.

To help in the planning of diets which would guarantee adequate nutrition for normal people, the U.S. Department of Agriculture has developed a method in which foods are classified into groups according to their similarity in nutrient content. This method enables consumers to select foods from given groups rather than having to calculate the amount of each nutrient individually. Originally there were eleven food groups. To make them easier to remember, the number of groups was reduced to seven (the "Basic Seven") and finally to five (the "Basic Four," plus "extras").

"Balancing" Your Diet

To get the amounts and kinds of nutrients you need, your daily average should include:

1. Fruits and/or vegetables and/or fruit juices: four servings, at least one of which is fresh or fresh-frozen and uncooked. Wide variety is desirable since vitamin content varies within this group.
2. Grains and/or grain products, including cereals, breads, rice, macaroni, etc.: four servings.
3. Meats and/or meat products, fish and/or poultry and/or eggs: two servings. Proteins, iron and niacin are "leader" nutrients in this group, so it also includes nuts and dried beans (legumes).
4. Milk and/or milk products: two to four servings (with less needed as one grows up).

These groups are known as the "four basics" or "Basic Four." An easy way to remember them is to think of a cheeseburger with lettuce and tomato. It has them all (although some varieties may be too fatty to recommend them for a steady diet). In addition to the four basics, there is a fifth category, "extras," which includes fats, oils, sugar and alcohol. These add variety and calories, and should be taken in moderation. Fats and oils also provide essential fatty acids. ("Essential" means needed in the diet because the body cannot make it in adequate amounts or at all.)

Food classifications and serving sizes are defined in the *Daily Food Guide* published by the Agriculture Department (see Appendix B). Eight ounces of milk, 2-3 ounces of meat, ½ cup of vegetables and one slice of bread are examples of serving sizes. Adhering literally to the minimum servings recommended in the food guide will provide about 1,200 calories and adequate amounts of all essential amino acids, fatty acids, vitamins and minerals. Since most people eat more than this, it should be clear that eating a wide variety of foods from the Basic Four will easily provide you with all the nutrients you need, even if some of the foods are not rich in nutrients. *Rather than promoting the Basic Four, vitamin hustlers teach "nutrition insurance" with unnecessary supplements.*

Vitamin Facts

A vitamin is an organic (carbon-containing) molecule needed in the diet in tiny amounts. Continued lack of any vitamin in an otherwise complete diet will result in a deficiency disease, the best known of which are beriberi, pellagra, rickets and scurvy. Vitamins were first discovered by investigators searching for the cause of these diseases.

Thirteen substances are vitamins for humans. Four are fat-soluble (A, D, E and K) and nine are water-soluble (C and the eight "B-complex" vitamins: thiamin, riboflavin, niacin, B_6, pantothenic acid, B_{12}, biotin and folic acid). It is unlikely that any new vitamins will be found. The last one was discovered in 1948, and three decades of intensive research have not uncovered any more. Moreover, patients have now lived quite well for years on just intravenous solutions which contain the known nutrients. If there were an undiscovered vitamin, these patients would have shown evidence of a deficiency disease.

Vitamins can function in the body in two ways. In small amounts, they function as *catalysts*. A catalyst is a substance that increases the speed of a chemical reaction without being used up by the reaction. Vitamins help accelerate certain chemical reactions that are essential for health. Without vitamins, these reactions would occur very slowly or not at all. The fact that vitamins are not used up explains why they are needed in only tiny amounts. Amounts of vitamins beyond what the body needs do not function usefully as vitamins but act like *chemicals* or *drugs*. Excesses of water-soluble vitamins are excreted in the urine. Fat-soluble vitamins, particularly A and D, are potentially more dangerous because they accumulate in body fat. Even modest excesses can build up gradually over months or years to toxic levels.

To clarify in your mind why extra vitamins are not needed, imagine you are hovering in the sky over an intersection (vitamin receptor site) where one police officer (vitamin) at a time is enough to insure that automobile traffic (food) will flow smoothly. Although many cars pass through the intersection (get "used up"), the police officers will need only an occasional replacement when they go off-duty. Bringing more police officers (excess vitamins) to the intersection will not improve the flow of traffic. It will merely add to taxpayer expense.

The rapid excretion of excess water-soluble vitamins can be demonstrated by a simple test. Riboflavin, for which the adult RDA is about 1.6 mg, has a bright yellow color. Swallow 2-3 vitamin pills which give you a total of 5 mg of riboflavin. Wait an hour and urinate. The reason why Americans have the most expensive urine and the best-nourished toilets in the world will then be obvious.

To promote vitamin supplements, health hustlers misrepresent the concept of "biochemical individuality" to imply that individuals should consume more than the RDAs in case they have greater-than-average nutrient needs. We have already mentioned that RDAs are deliberately set considerably higher than most people require in order to encompass the range of individual variations. In other words, biochemical individuality *has* been taken into account. Moreover, if individual variation were as great as the hustlers would have us believe, it would also apply to the inability to tolerate higher doses of nutrients—extra nutrients would be as likely to make people sick as they would be to help them.

There are only two situations in which the use of vitamins in excess of the RDAs is legitimate. The first is for treatment of *medically diagnosed* deficiency states—conditions which are rare except among alcoholics, persons with intestinal absorption defects, and the poor, especially those who are pregnant or elderly. The other use is in treatment of certain conditions for which large doses of vitamins are being used experimentally as drugs—with full recognition of the risks involved.

The Danger of Excess Vitamins

Many substances which are harmless in small or moderate doses can be harmful in large amounts or by gradual build-up over many years. Just because a substance (such as a vitamin) is found naturally in food does not mean that it cannot be harmful. In fact, an entire book has been written on this subject: *Toxicants Occurring Naturally in Foods, 2nd Edition*, published by a subcommittee of the National Research Council. The book includes a chapter on the toxicity of vitamins.

Megadoses of almost every nutrient have been demonstrated to be harmful. Too much vitamin A can cause lack of appetite, retarded growth in children, drying and cracking of the skin, enlargement of the liver and spleen, increased pressure on the brain, loss of hair, migratory joint pains, menstrual difficulty, bone pain, irritability and headache.

Prolonged excessive intake of vitamin D can cause loss of appetite, nausea, weakness, weight loss, excess urinary output, constipation, vague aches, stiffness, kidney stones, tissue calcification, high blood pressure, acidosis and kidney failure which can lead to death.

Large doses of niacin, as recommended by purveyors of megavitamins for mental disorders, can cause severe flushing, itching, liver damage, skin disorders, gout, ulcers and blood sugar disorders.

Excess vitamin E can cause headaches, nausea, tiredness, giddiness, inflammation of the mouth, chapped lips, gastrointestinal disturbances, muscle weakness, low blood sugar, increased bleeding tendency and degenerative changes. By antagonizing the action of vitamin A, large doses of vitamin E can cause blurred vision. Vitamin E can also reduce sexual organ function—just the opposite of the false claim that the vitamin heightens sexual potency. (This claim is based on fertility experiments with rats. Quacks don't tell you that what may be true with rats may be just the opposite with man!)

Another way to look for health trouble is with large doses of ascorbic acid—vitamin C. Here the quacks take great pleasure in linking themselves with one of the truly great men of our age, Linus Pauling, who won Nobel Prizes for chemistry in 1954 and for peace in 1962. Pauling's belief that vitamin C has value against the common cold may have slight validity, but its value is quite limited. Like an antihistamine tablet, in some cases it may reduce the symptoms of a mild cold (thereby creating the impression that no cold occurred). There is no reliable evidence that large doses of vitamin C *prevent* colds, and it is therefore not logical to take such doses 365 days a year.

Evidence has been published that under certain circumstances, large doses of vitamin C can damage vitamin B_{12} status. In fact, megadoses of vitamin C may convert some B_{12} to anti-B_{12} molecules. In addition, excess vitamin C may damage growing bone, produce diarrhea, produce "rebound scurvy" in adults and in newborn infants whose mothers took large doses, cause adverse effects in pregnancy, produce kidney stones and cause false urine tests for sugar in diabetes. Vitamin C in large doses can also produce false negative tests for blood in the stool and thereby prevent early detection of serious gastrointestinal diseases including cancer.

Adverse effects such as those listed above are unlikely to occur with water-soluble vitamins at intake levels below 10 times the RDAs, or with fat-soluble vitamins below 3 times the RDAs. But even if lesser dosages don't harm you physically, if you don't need them, they are a waste of money.

Mineral Facts

The important minerals known to be essential to man are calcium, phosphorus, magnesium and the trace elements: iron, zinc, copper, manganese, fluoride, chromium, selenium and molybdenum. Like fat-soluble vitamins, excess amounts of minerals are stored in the body and can gradually build up to toxic levels. An excess of one mineral can also interfere with the functioning of others. There are legitimate reasons for certain people to use mineral supplements, but they should never be used without medical supervision.

Iron is needed for blood formation, and new blood is formed rapidly in three groups: children up to age 5, boys and girls at the onset of puberty, and women who must replace blood lost during menstruation. Vegetarians must be particularly careful because vegetable iron is much less absorbable than is iron from animal sources. Iron deficiency is common enough in these groups that they should be evaluated with a blood test for iron deficiency. If it is found, treatment with iron should be administered. Taking iron if you don't have proven iron deficiency is unwise, since it can produce iron overload that can damage the liver, pancreas and heart.

Fluoride is needed to help form teeth that are strong and resistant to decay. Children whose community water supplies are not fluoridated should take a daily fluoride supplement up to the age of 12. Except for iron and fluoride, there is little likelihood of mineral deficiency developing in anyone who eats a balanced diet.

Zinc deficiency may occur in people whose diets are unbalanced with too much fiber (vegetarian diets) because fiber can pull zinc out of the food and into the stool. This can occur even when zinc is eaten in RDA amounts. One portion of meat a day satisfies most mineral requirements.

As with vitamins, the best way to avoid trouble with minerals is to obtain them in the rational packages of nature—foods in a balanced diet.

This book describes how food quacks are selling the American public a bill of anti-scientific goods and what should be done about it.

Chapter 2

The Modern Food Quack

Most people think that quackery is easy to spot. It is not. The modern quack wears a cloak of science. He talks in "scientific" terms and writes with scientific references. He is introduced on talk shows as a "scientist ahead of his time." He may indeed appear to be an expert.

The very word "quack" helps his camouflage by making us think of an outlandish character selling snake oil from the back of a covered wagon—and of course intelligent people wouldn't buy snake oil nowadays, would they?

Well, snake oil isn't selling so well lately. But vitamins? Minerals? "Organic" foods? Stress formulas? Tonics? Oral enzymes? The latest diet book? Herbal remedies? Bee pollen? Ginseng? Hair analysis? B_{15}? Laetrile? Systems to "balance body chemistry"? Megavitamins for mental illness? Or B_{12} shots to pep you up? Business is booming for the food quack. His annual take is in the *billions!*

What sells is not the quality of his products but the quack's ability to influence his audience. To those in pain, he promises relief. To the incurable, he offers hope. To the nutrition-conscious, he says, "Make sure you have enough." To a public worried about pollution, he says, "Buy natural." To one and all, he promises better health and a longer life. The modern quack has learned to reach people on the level that counts the most.

How can we tell the difference between a nutrition expert and a food quack? Here are 17 tips to help you identify a quack:

1. He advises you to buy something which you would not otherwise have bought.

He tells you all the wonderful things that vitamins, minerals and other nutrients do in your body, and what can happen if you don't get enough. But he conveniently neglects to tell you that deficiences are rare, that eating a balanced diet will give you all the nutrients you need, and that balancing your diet is simple. Nor does he tell you that nutrients are sufficiently plentiful that all but the most outlandish sorts of diets will give you enough of them. He wants you to think that "more is better," and that the expensive supplements and health foods he promotes are vital for your health.

2. He says that most disease is due to a faulty diet.

This is not so. Ask your doctor or inspect any medical school textbook of medicine. They will tell you that most diseases have nothing to do with diet. Common symptoms like malaise (feeling poorly), tiredness, lack of pep, aches (including headaches) or pains, insomnia and similar complaints, are usually the body's reaction to emotional stress, overwork, etc. The persistence of such symptoms is not a reason to add vitamins. It is a reason to see a doctor to be evaluated for possible underlying physical illness.

3. He suggests that most people are poorly nourished.

This is an appeal to fear which is not only untrue, but ignores the fact that the main forms of poor nourishment in the United States are undernourishment in the poverty-stricken and overweight in the economically well-to-do. The poverty-stricken can ill afford to waste money on unnecessary vitamins. Their food money should be spent for nourishing food.

It is being alleged that modern advertising has produced widespread addiction to "junk" foods, making a well-rounded diet exceptional rather than usual. The first part of this charge may be true, but the second part is not. It is true that some snack foods are mainly "empty calories" (sugars and/or fats without other nutrients). But it is not necessary for every morsel of food we eat to be loaded with nutrients. The small amounts of vitamins and minerals that our bodies require are easily obtained by eating a balanced variety of foods, and most "fast foods" contain substantial amounts of vitamins and minerals.

Most vitamin pushers suggest that everyone is in danger of vitamin deficiency. Here are two examples, one from the flyer of a prominent supermarket chain and the other from a major department store chain:

No matter how hard you try, in our fast food society, it's often difficult to make sure you're getting enough essential vitamins and minerals in the food you eat. When you remember that the health of your eyes depends upon a sufficient intake of these vital nutrients, it's hard not to see why neglect of them in your diet can cause needless health problems. Vitamin and mineral supplements, included in your daily diet, can assure you that your body will maintain the level of organic compounds it needs, not only to transform food into energy, but to function properly.

Today's lifestyles, eating habits and processed foods may make it difficult for you to get the vitamins and nutrients your body needs every day to carry on normal cellular functions . . . Quite possibly deficiencies of many nutrients may be common. Of the approximately 40 nutrients that are considered elemental in meeting daily body requirements, many cannot be manufactured or stored by the body. These nutrients must be ingested daily. Regardless of age, sex, where you live or what you do, proper preventive self care may require the nutritional protection of daily dietary supplements.

Do these sound scary? They are meant to be. Their pitch is like that of the door-to-door furnace huckster who states that your perfectly good furnace is in danger of blowing up unless you replace it with his product.

Scientists sometimes use the term "subclinical deficiency" to refer to a person on the road to deficiency from an inadequate diet. But no normal person eating a well-balanced diet each day is in any danger of vitamin deficiency, subclinical or otherwise.

There is a form of poor nourishment which is particularly common in this country—fluoride deficiency. Fluoride is necessary to build strong teeth which resist decay. The best way for people to get enough of this essential nutrient is to adjust community water supplies so that they contain about one part fluoride for every million parts of water. The quack is usually opposed to water fluoridation and may use scare tactics to sell "purifiers" to remove fluoride from your drinking water. It almost seems that if he can't personally profit from the sale, he isn't interested in your health!

4. He tells you that soil depletion and the use of "chemical" fertilizers result in less nourishing food.

This claim is used to promote the sale of so-called "organic" foods (see Chapter 7). If a nutrient is missing from the soil, a plant just does not grow. Chemical fertilizers counteract the effects of soil depletion. Plants do vary in mineral content, but this is rarely significant in the diet. The quack is dead wrong when he claims otherwise! He is also wrong when he claims that plants grown with natural fertilizers (such as manure) are nutritionally superior to those grown with synthetic fertilizers. Before using them, plants convert natural fertilizers into the same chemicals that synthetic fertilizers supply. The only "extra" you may get from animal fertilizer is a good case of *Salmonella* diarrhea or intestinal parasites. Moreover, "natural" foods are more likely to have molds growing on them which produce potent carcinogens (cancer-producers) called aflatoxins. Some food additives reduce the growth of molds.

5. He claims that modern processing methods and storage remove all nutritive value from our food.

This is a gross exaggeration of fact. It is true that food processing can change the nutrient contents of foods. But the changes are not so drastic as the quack, who wants you to buy his supplements, would like you to believe. While some processing methods destroy nutrients, others add them. So long as you select your foods daily from all four basic food groups (grain, meat, milk, and fruit and vegetable), you will get all the nourishment you need.

The quack distorts and oversimplifies. When he states that milling removes B vitamins, he does not bother to tell you that enrichment, *required by law,* puts them back. When he says that cooking destroys vitamins, he does not tell you that only a few of them are sensitive to heat. Nor does he tell you that these vitamins are easily obtained by having just one portion of fresh fruit or vegetable or fruit juice each day. Any claims that minerals are destroyed by processing or cooking are pure lies. Heat does not destroy minerals.

6. He tells you that under stress, and in certain diseases, your need for nutrients is increased.

An increasing number of major pharmaceutical companies have been using these tactics lately. One company asserts that "if you drink, smoke, diet, or happen to be sick, you may be robbing your body of vitamins." Another warns that "stress can deplete your body of water-soluble vitamins . . . and daily replacement is necessary." Another plugs its product to fill the "special needs of athletes."

While it is true that the need for vitamins may rise slightly under stress and in certain diseases, these ads are misleading because the need almost never rises above the Recommended Dietary Allowance (RDA). The average American, stressed or not, is simply not in imminent danger of scurvy or beriberi. The increased needs referred to in the ads are neither significant nor unmet by proper eating. Someone who is really in danger of deficiency as a result of illness would be a very ill person who needs medical care, probably in a hospital. But these promotions are aimed at well-nourished members of the general public who certainly do not need vitamin supplements to survive the common cold, a round of golf, or a jog around the neighborhood!

The concept and formulation for these products appears to be adapted largely from a 1952 report on therapeutic nutrition, written by two scientists, which was issued by the National Academy of Science. The Academy subsequently issued a 3-page document recalling the report and asking libraries to remove it from their shelves because it was based on inadequate evidence—and that there is no justification for substantial dosage increase in "stress."

Advertising to health professionals and the general public suggests that smokers need extra vitamin C and women taking birth control pills need extra folic acid and vitamin B_{12}. While it is true that such people may have lower blood levels of these vitamins, these lower levels are still within the normal range. In the case of vitamin C, the levels of smokers are still 10 times deficiency levels. In America, cigarette smoking is the leading cause of death preventable by self-discipline. Rather than seeking false comfort by taking vitamin C, smokers who are concerned about their health should stop smoking.

7. He says you are in danger of being poisoned by food additives and preservatives.

This is a scare tactic designed to undermine your confidence in food scientists and government protection agencies. The quack wants you to think that *he* is out to protect you. He hopes that if you trust him, you will buy what he recommends. The fact is that the tiny amounts of preservatives used to protect our food pose no threat to human health.

This chapter cannot cover this subject in detail, but we would like to point out how ridiculous quacks can get about food additives, especially some which are found naturally in food. Calcium propionate, which is used to preserve bread, occurs naturally in Swiss cheese. The quack who would steer you toward (higher-priced) bread made without preservatives is careful not to tell you that one ounce of Swiss cheese, which you may eat in a sandwich, contains enough calcium propionate to retard spoilage of two loaves of bread. Similarly, the quack who warns against monosodium glutamate (MSG) does not tell you that wheat germ is a major natural source of this substance.

Also curious is the fact that many plant substances sold in health food stores are potentially toxic and some can even cause death. About 30 such products, most of them herbal teas, are listed in Appendix A of this book.

8. He says that if you eat badly, you'll be OK if you take a vitamin or vitamin-mineral supplement.

This is the "Nutrition Insurance Gambit." It is dangerous nonsense. Not only is it untrue, but it encourages careless eating habits. The cure for eating badly is eating better. Money spent for a vitamin or mineral supplement would be better spent for a daily portion of fresh fruit, vegetable, milk, grain or meat product.

9. He recommends that everybody take vitamins or health foods or both.

The food quack belittles normal foods and ridicules the "basic four" of good nutrition. He may not tell you how he earns his living from such pronouncements—via public appearance fees, product endorsements, sale of publications or financial interests in vitamin companies, health food stores and/or organic farms. The very term "health food" is deceptive. Most regular foods are full of nutrients. Did you ever stop to think that your corner grocery, fruit market, meat market and supermarket are also health food stores? They are—and they usually charge less for food that is identical or superior to that provided by "health food" stores.

The quack often makes nutritional claims for bioflavonoids, rutin, inositol, para-aminobenzoic acid (PABA) and other such food substances. These "non-essential" ingredients are not needed in your diet, and the FDA forbids nutritional claims for them in labeling. When the quack calls them "vitamins," he does not tell you that they are vitamins for *bacteria*, not for *humans*. They won't help *you*, but PABA can help the growth of certain bacterial infections.

By the way, have you ever wondered why people who eat lots of "health foods" still feel they must load themselves up with vitamin supplements?

10. He recommends a wide variety of substances similar to those found in your body.

The underlying idea—reminiscent of the wishful thinking of primitive tribes—is that taking these substances will strengthen or rejuvenate body processes that involve similar substances. For example, according to a health food brochure:

> Raw glandular therapy, or "cellular therapy"—as it is called in Europe—seems almost too simple to be true. It consists of giving in supplemental form (intravenous or oral) those specific tissues from animals that correspond to the weakened areas of the human body. In other words, if a person has a weak pancreas, give him raw pancreas substance; if the heart is weak, give raw heart, etc.

The quack doesn't tell you that when these substances are taken by mouth, they are digested and destroyed by the stomach and intestines. In mainland China, powdered bull penis is sold as a remedy for male impotence.

Vitamins and minerals may be added to the various preparations. When taken by mouth, such preparations are unlikely to do direct harm, but their promotion by the health food industry encourages extreme degrees of self-diagnosis and self-treatment. When injected, however, raw animal tissues can cause allergic reactions to their proteins; and some preparations have caused serious infections. Repeated injections can produce fatal allergic reactions.

Proponents of "tissue salts" suggest that the basic cause of disease is mineral deficiency—correction of which will enable the body to heal itself. Under this system of healing, one or more of 12 salts is appropriate for the prevention and treatment of a wide variety of diseases, including appendicitis (ruptured or not), baldness, deafness, insomnia and worms. Development of this method is attributed to a 19th century physician named W. H. Schuessler.

Enzymes for oral use are another ripoff. They supposedly can aid digestion and "support" many other functions within the body. The fact is, however, that enzymes taken by mouth are broken down into their component amino acids by digestion in the stomach and intestines and therefore do not even function as enzymes within the body. Pancreatic enzymes have some legitimate medical uses in diseases which are accompanied by decreased secretion of pancreatic enzymes into the intestine, but these diseases are not appropriate for self-diagnosis or self-treatment. Anyone who actually has a pancreatic enzyme deficiency may have a serious underlying disease that should be medically diagnosed and treated.

RNA (ribonucleic acid), another compound we produce in our bodies, is part of the reproductive apparatus of all cells. It is being promoted as a food supplement and as a factor in certain diets which supposedly can increase energy and make people look younger and healthier. When taken by mouth, RNA is broken down by a pancreatic enzyme and doesn't even get into the cells of the body—but one of its breakdown products can produce a dangerous elevation of the blood uric acid level. Moreover, RNA, like a photographic negative, is a specific blueprint. If RNA from yeasts or sardines could actually work in humans, it would turn them into young yeasts or baby sardines.

11. He claims that "natural" vitamins are better than "synthetic" ones.

This claim is a flat lie and anyone who makes it should be immediately classified by you as a quack. Each vitamin is a chain of atoms strung together as a molecule. Molecules made in the "factories" of nature are identical to those made in the factories of chemical companies. Does it make sense to pay extra for vitamins extracted from foods when you can get all you need from the foods themselves?

12. He warns that sugar is a "deadly poison."

Many recent books and magazine articles would have us believe that sugar is "the killer on the breakfast table" and is the underlying cause of everything from heart disease to hypoglycemia. The facts, however, are as follows:

1. When sugar is used in moderation as part of a normal, balanced diet, it is perfectly safe. Indeed, if you ate no sugar, your liver would make it because your brain requires it.
2. Sugar does not cause diabetes, even in excess amounts. (High levels may worsen this disease, however.)
3. Although sugar is a factor in the tooth decay process, what counts is not merely the amount of sugar in the diet but the length of time that *any* digestible carbohydrate remains in contact with the teeth (and the extent of oral hygiene practiced).
4. There is no evidence that sugar increases your chance of developing heart disease.
5. Sugar is not the cause of obesity. Overweight is caused by eating more calories than are used up in body activity. Excess calories will cause overweight regardless of what kind of food they are in.
6. Hypoglycemia ("low blood sugar") which is *rare*, is not caused by sugar.

13. He tells you it is easy to lose weight.

Diet quacks would have us believe that special combinations of foods or food supplements can be of great help to dieters. But the only way to lose weight is to burn off more calories than you eat. This requires self-discipline: eating less, exercising more, or preferably doing both. There are 3,500 calories in a pound of human fat. To lose one pound a week, you must eat an average of 500 fewer calories per day than you burn up. The most sensible diet for losing weight is one that is nutritionally balanced in carbohydrates, fats and proteins. Most fad diets, if followed closely, will result in weight loss—as a result of calorie restriction. But they are invariably too monotonous and are often dangerous for long-term use. Unless a dieter develops better eating habits, weight lost on a fad diet will soon return.

The term "cellulite" is sometimes used to describe the dimpled fat found on the hips and thighs of many women. Although no medical evidence supports the claim, cellulite is promoted as a special type of fat which is resistant to diet and exercise. Sure-fire cellulite remedies include creams (to "dissolve" it), brushes, rollers, "loofah" sponges, rubberized pants and vitamin-mineral supplements with herbs. The cost of various treatment plans runs from $10 for a bottle of vitamins to $500 or more at a salon that offers heat treatments, massage, enzyme injections and/or treatment with various gadgets. The simple truth about "cellulite" is that it doesn't exist—it is ordinary fat which can only be lost as part of an overall reducing program.

14. He promises quick, dramatic, miraculous cures.

The promises are usually subtle or couched in doubletalk—so he can deny making them when the feds close in. Such promises are the health hustler's most immoral practice. He does not want to know how many people have been broken financially or in spirit—by the elation over his claims of quick cure followed by deep depression when the claims prove false. Nor does the quack keep count of how many people he lures away from proper medical care.

Quacks will tell you that "megavitamins" (huge doses of vitamins) can cure many different ailments, particularly emotional ones. But they won't tell you that the "evidence" supporting such claims is unreliable because it is based on inadequate investigations, anecdotes or testimonials. Nor do quacks inform you that megadoses may be harmful. Megavitamin therapy is nutritional roulette.

Ginseng, described by a major promoter as "one of the most lucrative cash crops known to man," is claimed to be a healthful tonic and sexual enhancer. It is also being used to get "high" (*naturally*, of course!). But before you try it, take heed. It contains a variety of potentially toxic chemicals, some of which act like steroid drugs. Among its toxic effects are diarrhea, skin eruptions, insomnia, nervousness and severe mental confusion. Ginseng also contains small amounts of estrogens and has been reported to cause swollen and painful breasts.

15. He uses anecdotes and testimonials to support his claims.

We all tend to believe what others tell us about their personal experiences. But separating cause and effect from coincidence is not simple. When someone tells you that product X has cured his cancer, arthritis or whatever, be skeptical. He may not have actually had the condition he names. If he did have the condition, his recovery most likely would have occurred without the help of product X. Most single episodes of disease recover with just the passage of time, and most chronic ailments have symptom-free periods. Establishing medical truths requires careful and repeated investigation—with well-designed experiments, not reports of what people *imagine* might have taken place. That is why testimonial evidence is forbidden in scientific articles and is usually inadmissible in court.

The extent to which people can be fooled should not be underestimated. During the early 1940's, many thousands of people became convinced that a remedy promoted by William Koch, M.D., Ph.D., could cure cancer. Yet analysis of the product showed it to be distilled water! Many years before that, when arsenic was used as a "tonic," countless numbers of people swore by it even as it slowly poisoned them.

Symptoms which are psychosomatic (bodily reactions to tension) are often relieved by *any* product taken with a suggestion that it will work. Tiredness and other minor aches and pains will often respond to any enthusiastically recommended nostrum. For these problems, even physicians may prescribe a placebo. A placebo is a substance which has no pharmacological effect on a normal person, but is given to satisfy a patient who supposes it to be a medicine. Sugar tablets and vitamins (such as B_{12}) are commonly used in this way.

Placebos act by suggestion. Unfortunately, some physicians, like most laypersons, really "believe in vitamins" beyond those supplied by a good diet. Those who share such beliefs do so because they confuse placebo action with cause and effect.

Talk show hosts give quacks a tremendous boost when they ask them, "What do all the vitamins you take do for you personally?" Then millions of viewers are treated to the quack's talk of improved health, vigor and vitality—with the implicit point: "It did this for me. It will do the same for you."

A most revealing testimonial experience was described several years ago during a major network talk show which hosted several of the world's most prominent promoters of nutritional faddism. While the host was boasting about how his new eating program had cured his "hypoglycemia," he mentioned in passing that he no longer was drinking "20 to 30 cups of coffee a day." Neither the host nor any of his "experts" had the good sense to tell their audience how dangerous it can be to drink so much coffee. Nor did any of them suggest that most of the host's original symptoms were probably caused by caffeine intoxication. The average brewed cup of coffee contains 100 mg of caffeine, a significant dose. Excess amounts of caffeine can cause nervousness, irritability, insomnia, heart palpitations and gastrointestinal symptoms.

16. He'll offer you a vitamin that isn't.

Ernst T. Krebs, M.D., and his son, Ernst T. Krebs, Jr., patented an undefined mixture which they later trade-named "pangamate" and "vitamin B_{15}." The Krebs' are also the modern promoters of the ancient quack cancer remedy, amygdalin, which they first trade-named "laetrile" and now call "vitamin B_{17}."

To be a vitamin, a substance must be an organic nutrient which is necessary in the diet in small amounts; and deficiency of the substance must be shown to cause a specific disease. Neither pangamate nor laetrile is a vitamin. Laetrile contains 6 percent cyanide by weight; and it has poisoned people. Everyone who takes it gets at least low-grade cyanide poisoning which can be determined by measuring blood cyanide levels.

Pangamate is not even a single substance but is merely a label applied to differing product mixtures marketed by various manufacturers. Recent experiments have shown that ingredients in some of the most widely sold "pangamates" can cause mutations in bacteria—which means they may cause cancer in humans. Federal courts in Chicago, Pittsburgh and New Jersey have ordered three major manufacturers to stop marketing "vitamin B_{15}" products. In two of the cases, the judge ruled that the products were adulterated because they contained an unsafe food additive. In the third, the defendant signed a consent agreement to the same effect.

17. He espouses the "Conspiracy Theory" and its twin, the "Controversy Claim."

The quack claims he is being persecuted by orthodox medicine and that his work is being suppressed. He claims that orthodox medicine or the AMA is against him because his cures can cut into the incomes that doctors make by keeping people sick. He doesn't tell you that his own income may be much higher than that of orthodox physicians.

Don't fall for such nonsense! There is so much more medical business than American physicians can handle that we import large numbers of doctors each year. Moreover, many doctors in private or governmental health plans receive the same salary whether or not the patients in the plans are sick—so keeping their patients healthy reduces their workload but not their incomes.

Any physician who found a vitamin or other preparation which could cure sterility, heart disease, arthritis, cancer or the like, could make an enormous fortune from such a discovery. Not only would patients flock to him (as they now do toward anyone who falsely claims to cure such problems), but his colleagues would shower him with prizes—including the $200,000+ Nobel Prize! And don't forget, doctors get sick and so do their families. Do you believe that legitimate doctors would conspire to suppress cures for diseases which also afflict themselves and their loved ones?

The quack claims there is a "controversy" about facts between himself and "the bureaucrats," organized medicine and/or "the establishment." He clamors for medical investigation of "his" claims (ignoring the negative results of all past investigations). In reality, there is no factual controversy. The collision is between the quack's misleading statements and the facts. The gambit, "Do you believe in vitamins?" is another tactic he uses to increase confusion. Everyone knows that vitamins are needed by our bodies. The real question is "Do you need additional vitamins beyond those in a well-balanced diet?" The answer is NO. Nutrition is a science, not a religion. It is based upon matters of fact, not questions of *belief*.

This chapter does not mean to imply that everyone who promotes unnecessary nutrients is deliberately trying to mislead you. One reason why quackery is so difficult to spot is that most people who spread nutrition misinformation are quite sincere in their beliefs. Even if you keep the above list of 17 tips in mind, you still may be vulnerable to a sales pitch from someone you would never suspect.

Chapter 3

Friendly Salespeople

Most people who think they have been helped by vitamins enjoy sharing success stories with their friends. People who give such testimonials are usually motivated by a sincere desire to help others. Rarely do they stop to consider how serious it can be to make health recommendations to others. Nor do they realize how difficult it is to evaluate health products on the basis of personal experience. The average person who feels better after using a product cannot rule out coincidence (whether he would have felt better anyway) or the placebo effect (feeling better because he thinks he has taken a positive step). Since we all tend to believe what others tell us about personal experiences, testimonials can be powerful persuaders.

Three giant companies which sell food supplements are systematically turning their customers into salesmen. The Shaklee Corporation, which is based in San Francisco, claims to have "hundreds of thousands" of distributors. Its reported gross income in 1980 was $411,331,000, about two-thirds of it from the sale of nutritional products. The Neo-Life Company of America, headquartered in Hayward, California, has more than 100,000 distributors located primarily in the Western United States. Its 1980 gross income, though not publicly reported, was probably well over $200,000,000, with 70 percent of it from the sale of vitamins.

The Amway Corporation, of Ada, Michigan, claims to have more than 750,000 distributors worldwide. This company markets many types of household products in addition to nutrients. It also owns the Mutual (radio) Broadcasting System (which carries the questionable nutrition advice of Carlton Fredericks). Amway's reported 1980 gross income was $825,000,000, about 20 percent of which was from the sale of food supplements from its Nutrilite Division. These figures indicate that *retail* sales of food supplements in 1980 by these three companies together exceeded $700,000,000!

Becoming a salesman for these companies is quite simple and requires no prior knowledge of nutrition. Many people do so initially in order to buy their own supplements at a discount. For small sums of money ($12.50 for Shaklee, $20 for Neo-Life, $64 for Amway), the companies will sell you a distributor's kit which includes promotional literature, price lists, order forms and a detailed instructional manual. Each also provides a monthly magazine which contains company philosophy, product news, success stories and photographs of top salespeople.

"When you share our products," says the Shaklee sales manual, "you're not just selling. You're passing on news about products you believe in to people you care about. Make a list of people you know; you'll be surprised how long it will be. This is your first list of potential customers." The goal is not merely to sell products, but to encourage your more enthusiastic customers to become salesmen themselves.

"Recruiting is the lifeblood of your business," the Neo-Life manual points out. "If you believe that our company is the greatest in the world, if you believe that your products are the finest products you have ever discovered or used, and if you believe the opportunity is the greatest financial opportunity in the world— then your conviction, belief and excitement will make you a good recruiter, providing you share your conviction with everyone you meet." The more you sell, the more salemen you recruit and supervise, the higher your profit percentages and bonuses. Top-flight sales leaders can earn a car allowance, free vacation trips and more than $100,000 a year while "working to benefit humanity." Those who work out of their homes can also deduct certain household expenses as business deductions.

At least four smaller supplement companies—Sunasu, Forever Living, Pro-Vita and Enhance—have similar "pyramidal" marketing structures. Enhance was formed in 1979 by Robert J. Wooten, former $150,000-a-year board chairman of Shaklee Corporation. Sales of Enhance products passed $1 million a month within a year and are expected to hit $3-5 million a month by the end of 1981. A recent article in *Health Foods Business* estimates that person-to-person sales of food supplements will exceed one *billion* dollars in 1981. The article's author, a former health food store owner, suggests that store owners "fight fire with fire" by recruiting their own door-to-door sales forces.

The Story of Nutrilite

The concept of Nutrilite is said to have originated about 50 years ago in the mind of Carl Rehnborg, an American businessman who lived in China from 1917 to 1927. According to Amway publications, this gave Rehnborg "ample opportunity to observe at close range the effects of inadequate diet." He also "became familiar with the nutritional literature of his day." Concluding that a balanced diet was needed for proper bodily function, he began to envision a dietary supplement which could provide people with important nutrients regardless of their eating habits.

After seven years of "experimentation," Rehnborg produced food supplements which he gave to his friends to try. According to his son, Sam, who is now Nutrilite's executive vice president and director of research:

> After a certain length of time, Dad would visit his friends to see what results had been obtained. More often than not, he would find the products sitting on the back shelves, unused and forgotten. It had cost them nothing and was therefore, to them, worth nothing . . . It was at this point that he rediscovered a basic principle—that the answer was merely to charge something for the product. When he did, the friends, having paid for the product, ate it, liked it, and further, wanted their friends to have it also. When they asked my dad to sell the product to their friends, he said, "You sell it to them and I'll pay you a commission."

Carl Rehnborg's food supplement business, which thus began as the California Vitamin Corporation, changed its name to Nutrilite Products in 1939 when it moved to larger quarters.

According to Federal District Court records, significant out-of-state distribution of Nutrilite supplements began in 1945 when a company operated by Lee S. Mytinger and William S. Casselberry became exclusive national distributor. Rehnborg acted as "scientific advisor" in the distributional scheme and would explain to sales groups that his supplements contained a secret base of unusual therapeutic value and were the answer to man's search for health.

Gross sales soared to $500,000 a month, but the promoters also ran afoul of the law. In 1947, the U.S. Food and Drug Administration (FDA) began a 4-year struggle to force Mytinger, Casselberry, Rehnborg, their respective companies and some 15,000 door-to-door agents to stop making wild claims about their products. Potential customers were being given a booklet, *How to Get Well and Stay Well*, which represented Nutrilite as effective against "almost every case" of allergies, asthma, mental depression, irregular heartbeat, tonsillitis and some 20 other common ailments. The booklet, which contained testimonial letters, also implied that cancer, heart trouble, tuberculosis, arthritis and many other serious illnesses would respond to Nutrilite treatment.

After Mytinger and Casselberry, Inc., was asked by the government to show cause why a criminal proceeding for misbranding should not be started, the booklet was revised. A "new language" was devised which referred to all diseases as "a state of non-health" brought about by a "chemical imbalance." Nutrilite would cure nothing—the patient merely gets well through its use. Most direct curative claims were removed from the booklet, but illustrative case histories were added. Although continued governmental pressure led to removal of the case histories, the booklet remained grossly misleading.

In 1951, the Court issued a permanent injunction forbidding anyone who sold Nutrilite products from referring to any edition of *How to Get Well and Stay Well* and more than 50 other publications which exaggerate the importance of food supplements. The court decree also contains a long list of forbidden and permissible claims about nutrition and Nutrilite products.

Today, although the origin of that list is not revealed, it is given to Nutrilite distributors almost in its entirety. Salesmen are not authorized by Amway to suggest, for example, that vitamin deficiencies are common, that faulty nutrition is the major cause of disease, or that food supplement use is likely to bring about a condition of health or prevent or cure any of a long list of serious diseases. The use of testimonials or personal experiences is also not authorized by Amway.

Nutrilite XX, the company's leading food supplement, contains 12 vitamins and 8 minerals, most in amounts approximating their recommended dietary allowances. A 1-month supply, which cost about $20 in 1950, now costs about $30. The current official sales pitch, simple and low-keyed, is based on the concepts of "subclinical deficiency" and "nutritional insurance" described in Chapter 2 of this book. Prospective customers are given a 60-page booklet, *Food and Your Family*, which explains the importance of nutrients, lists reasons why people's diets may be inadequate, and asks whether they think there is room for improvement in their own diet.

An FDA survey of health practices and opinions, conducted in 1969, shows quite clearly why this type of sales approach is bound to be successful. The survey found that most adults *mistakenly* believe that:

1. Extra vitamins will provide more pep and energy.
2. People who feel tired and run down probably need more vitamins and minerals.
3. Most Americans do not eat balanced diets.

According to *Food and Your Family*, hundreds of thousands of Americans have used Nutrilite "morning, noon and night for more than 40 years." If this claim is accurate (which is questionable), most of these lucky customers would have spent close to $10,000 for their pills!

The Shaklee Way of Life

Shaklee Corporation was founded in 1956 by Forrest C. Shaklee, a retired chiropractor said to have a lifelong interest in "improving health by working with Nature." According to company literature, he was sickly at birth, but eventually "learned to overcome his deficiency with a program of exercise and nutrition."

During his teens, Shaklee became interested in the ideas of Bernarr Macfadden. In 1912, at the age of 18, he helped Macfadden tour midwestern cities to spark interest in "physical culture." According to the biography now sold by the Shaklee Corporation:

> Parades were held on the main street of each town, and consisted of a pride of muscular youths [including Shaklee], some musicians, and a flatbed wagon . . . When enough of a crowd had been gathered around the flatbed, each of the youths was to exercise with a given piece of equipment. This was preceded by a discourse by Macfadden, extolling health through nature, diet and especially non-diet (he tended to look upon fasting as a blanket cure-all) and, of course, strenuous exercise . . .
>
> The *piece-de-resistance* of these outdoor displays was the lifting of an iron ball which appeared to weigh easily 500 pounds. Secured to the ball was a massive link chain, which one of the youths would grasp and which, with much concentration and apparent straining, he would raise gradually over his head. The crowds, watching in awed silence at the beginning of the feat, would break into cheers and applause when the ball was finally lifted. When it was his turn at the ball, Forrest discovered that lifting it was easily accomplished; the ball was hollow!

Within the next few years, Shaklee graduated from chiropractic school and began to treat patients with a substance he developed and called "vitalized minerals." He then became head of several chiropractic clinics where he "concentrated on treating patients who had nutritional disorders." In the early 1940s, he stopped clincial practice but continued to lecture on nutrition. In 1956, he and his sons, Raleigh and Forrest, Jr., began marketing some of the products used by Shaklee during his practice. These products included *Pro-Lecin* (a combination of protein and lecithin), *Herb-Lax* (a herbal laxative) and *Vita-Lea* (a multiple vitamin-mineral supplement). Eventually a wide variety of other supplements, food products, cleaning products and cosmetics were added to the company line.

"Basic to the Shaklee Way of Life," says *The Shaklee Sales Manual,* is the belief that you have the right to prosper through your own personal efforts." Thousands of the company's distributors maintain a gross sales volume exceeding $3,000 a month.

The Shaklee sales approach is similar to that of Nutrilite, but some of its authorized practices are a bit more misleading. A section of the sales manual called "Appearances Can Deceive" suggests a variety of ways to make people worry that they are not getting enough nutrients in their food. The importance of each nutrient is described in detail, "individuality" of needs is stressed, and various situations are described wherein nutrients supposedly may be lacking. The fact that vitamin deficiency is *rare*, of course, is not mentioned.

The sales manual advises new distributors to sell to their friends "as a natural extension of your friendship." Other prospects can be contacted with a letter that begins: "Dear Mrs. Jones: Would you be interested in learning how you can simplify your shopping and at the same time provide total care for your family?" ("Total care," however, is not defined.)

Many Shaklee distributors appear to be making claims that go far beyond those authorized by the company. In 1981, Susan Fitzgerald and Pete Mekeel of *The Lancaster (Pa.) New Era* found that distributors in their county "tend to follow the example of their local leadership." The two reporters, who attended local sales meetings, observed a wide variety of testimonials being given for Shaklee products:

> People stand up at meetings and in the best spirit of an old-fashioned revival tell how Shaklee products have rid them of arthritis, saved their marriage, enabled them to have two bowel movements a day, and kept them from breaking a leg when they fell off a ladder. If there are any doubters, they keep quiet.

When the reporters consulted Shaklee distributors as potential clients, they were advised to buy a "Basic Five Plan" of supplements and *Herb-Lax* which would cost close to $600 per year per person.

Shaklee became a publicly owned corporation in 1973 and has been listed on the New York Stock Exchange since 1977. The company's 1980 annual report to the Securities and Exchange Commission indicates that on November 3, 1980, Forrest C. Shaklee, Jr., Raleigh L. Shaklee and their immediate families owned or held in trust 46.3 percent of the outstanding shares of stock—2,878,654 shares—whose market value was more than $62 million.

More Scare Tactics

Neo-Life Company of America was co-founded in 1958 by Donald F. Pickett, current chairman of its board of directors. Neo-Life publications describe him as a man who has been "deeply concerned about human survival in this over-chemicalized world," and who is also "nationally recognized as a nutritional expert." Although the publications do not describe Mr. Pickett's background or provide any basis for considering him a nutrition expert, they do spell out how to sell vitamins. One approach is the following:

Do you meet people who complain about being tired, sluggish or listless? Would they like to feel better, look better and have more energy? Maybe their nutritional fuel level is low, their diet is lacking in some essentials.

Ask them, "Would you put *used* motor oil in the engine of a brand new car?" Of course, they'll say no! We all know that the new car probably would perform fine—*for a while!* But, in the long run, the poor quality of the oil would *shorten* the life of the automobile and would *lower its performance!*

The body is no different! If you put junk food in it, it may perform trouble-free—for a while—but food low in nutrients will have the same long-term effects on the body as used oil does to the automobile—lower performance and greater wear and tear. And, unfortunately, you can't trade in on a new model when this one wears out! Remember, there's lots of "cheap fuel" around today; most packaged foods have many, if not all, of the natural nutrients removed during processing and replaced with chemicals.

Use this example when sharing Neo-Life nutritional products with your customers. They put *back* many of the essential vitamins and minerals that may be lacking in their diet today . . .

Most of your customers will say that they eat three balanced meals a day. Ask them if they are *sure* they are getting enough of the nutritional elements their bodies require . . . If there's any doubt, wouldn't they be willing to spend a few pennies a day to be sure?

Yes, even though "nutritional insurance" is rarely more valuable than insurance against a plague of unicorns, many people are willing to spend those "pennies." *Formula IV*, Neo-Life's multiple vitamin-mineral supplement, costs about 24¢ per day. If a potential customer says he can't afford this, the saleman is instructed to say, "Really, the only thing you have to decide is which of these *can* you afford: healthy cells, or weakened, sluggish cells."

For about $1 per day, customers can buy one of three *Uni-Pak* formulas that are "specifically tailored for their individual needs":

> *Exec 30* is a selection of supplements for office workers who find themselves desk-bound and sedentary, tired and listless.
>
> *Sports 30* is for customers of any age—from young adults active in sports to "on-the-go" active seniors . . . With *Sports 30* your customers will have the stamina and endurance to maintain an active pace. This carefully designed daily supplementation program provides vital nutrients required to help the body handle physical stress.
>
> *Stress 30* is for the decision-maker under pressure; housewife, foreman, student, truck driver—anyone with deadlines to meet—*Stress 30* helps you do it more and do it better. Your customers don't have to be high-powered executives; just about everyone faces tension or stress in day-to-day living. That means everyone you talk to is a potential customer.

To help potential customers estimate their stress levels, they may be given a "stress test" in which they check off items on a list of 43 causes of stress, each of which is assigned a point score from 11 to 100. Although this test may have some research applications in the field of psychology, it has nothing whatsoever to do with nutrient needs. But no matter, Neo-Life's Uni-Paks are "designed specifically to help *you* combat the effects of daily stress." Really? Like marriage (50 points), a mortgage over $10,000 (31 points) or outstanding personal achievement (28 points)?

If these products don't turn you on, how about some *Toxgard* to "help your body protect itself against heavy metal pollutants in air and water" and to "aid your liver in detoxifying food additives and artificial food colors." Or some *Liver Plus C*, on a hunch that "nutritionists believe that liver is a rich source of unknown nutritional factors which one day may be better known or appreciated."

Or some *Pet-Pal* to make your dog or cat less susceptible to "people" diseases? To become a customer for life, you don't have to fall for *all* of the claims promoted by supplement pushers. *Just one.*

A New Way of Life?

Imagine for a moment that you have been feeling lonely, bored, depressed or tired. One day a friend tells you that "improving your nutrition" can help you feel better. After selling you some vitamins, she inquires regularly to find out how you are doing. You seem to feel somewhat better. From time to time you are invited to interesting lectures where you meet people like yourself. Then you are asked to become a distributor. This keeps you busy, raises your family income, and provides an easy way to approach old friends and make new ones—all in an atmosphere of enthusiasm. Everybody helping everybody. Many of your customers express gratitude, giving you a feeling of accomplishment. You may even gain a free car, a mink coat and a trip to Hawaii!

Shaklee refers to this sales process as "sharing." Amway refers to it as "friends helping friends." Neo-Life calls it "A New Way of Life" and spells out the following benefits:

Relationships	Appreciation
Recognition	Excitement
Self Image	Adventure
Potential	Freedom
Income	Health

Is there anything wrong with feeling better the Neo-Life Way, the Shaklee Way or the Nutrilite Way?

We believe there is. First of all, the concept of "nutritional insurance" is a scare tactic. There are enough *real* things in life to worry about. Who needs imaginary ones?

Then there is the matter of money. Who needs to waste $30 or more per month buying an unnecessary product? Even if people insist on supplementing their diet for "insurance," there is no reason to spend more than a penny or two a day for a multivitamin-mineral supplement. The body cannot tell one brand from another. Nor is there ever any reason to buy a supplement which contains more than the RDA for any nutrient. If all supplement users were to limit themselves to RDA dosage at the lowest available cost, do you think the health food industry would survive?

There are also health risks associated with the taking of food supplements. Excess amounts of nutrients can harm people. Do you think that food supplement salespeople—many of whom believe that "more is better"—are qualified to judge how many pills per day their customers should take? Or which of their fatigued customers need medical care? Even though curative claims are forbidden by the written policies of each company, the sales process encourages customers to experiment with self-treatment. It also promotes distrust of legitimate health professionals and their treatment methods.

Some people would argue that the *apparent* benefits of "believing" in food supplements outweigh the risks involved. Do you think that people need false beliefs in order to feel healthy or succeed in life? Would you like to believe that something can help you when in fact it is worthless and may be harmful? Do you want our society to support an industry that is trying to mislead us? Can't Americans do something better with the billions of dollars being wasted each year on food supplements?

Chapter 4

Promises Everywhere

Suggestions to take vitamins seem to be everywhere. Advertisements on radio and television and in magazines and newspapers warn against deficiencies. Self-appointed "experts," echoed by a chorus of believers, praise the "miracles" of nutrition. Colorful bottles line the shelves—not only in health food stores but also in pharmacies, supermarkets and department stores. Doctors even prescribe vitamins as placebos. The great vitamin hustle now costs consumers more than two *billion* dollars a year.

Why do people take vitamins and how do they decide which ones to buy?

Most food supplement users believe they are getting "nutritional insurance," but the majority also believe that extra vitamins can give extra energy, improve general health and prevent disease. Consistent with these beliefs, most vitamin users take multivitamin or vitamin-mineral preparations. A smaller number of users believe that individual supplements can prevent or relieve specific ailments. The most popular individual supplements are vitamin C, vitamin E, and the B-vitamins, in that order. A recent survey found that multivitamin users are more likely to shop in pharmacies or supermarkets (where the prices are usually lower), while users of specific supplements are more likely to shop in health food stores or by mail.

It is obvious that most people who use *individual* supplements believe that these products have medicinal properties. This chapter illustrates some of the ways that such false beliefs are encouraged by health food store operators and various types of unlicensed "nutrition consultants." It also describes the marketing of herbs.

Industry Guidelines

A close look at food supplement bottles will show that almost none of them contains *therapeutic* claims on their labels. The reason for this is obvious. Unless a claim is backed by proof acceptable to the FDA (which simply means that there is reasonable evidence that it is true), it is illegal to make that claim on a label. Misbranded products can be seized and ultimately destroyed by government agencies. This means, incidentally, that if a health claim does not appear on a product's label or accompanying literature from its manufacturer, you can be sure the product won't do what is claimed.

It is also illegal for health food store operators to practice medicine without a license by diagnosing ailments or recommending that specific foods or food supplements be taken at specific times for specific ailments.

The National Nutritional Foods Association (NNFA), an organization of health food retailers, producers and distributors, has issued guidelines that provide "a reasonable and acceptable way to give nutritional advice to customers without prescribing." NNFA suggests that if a customer asks for advice about a specific ailment, the retailer should respond with a disclaimer. He should say that the store sells items for the building of health, rather than for the treatment of disease, and if the customer has a definite problem in mind, he should consult a physician. After doing this, the retailer can then redirect the discussion to "the relationship of better nutrition and a better state of health." (Do you think any such discussion will ever fail to recommend a product sold in the store?) If a customer asks about the efficacy of a particular item, the recommended answer is, "Yes, I have heard this, and many of our publications are available for your information." NNFA also warns retailers not to diagnose disease or advise customers to abandon their current medical care.

Similar advice is given from time to time in the trade magazine, *Health Foods Business*. A 1977 issue, for example, describes how a proprietor "keeps a couple of nutrition textbooks handy under the sales counter and when a question arises about the function or use of a product, he looks it up. He's very careful to stress that he is not a physician and that what he says should be taken as informative rather than authoritative." In a more recent issue, another storekeeper states:

> *We can avoid prescribing through the use of books . . .*
>
> In our stores we provide an area near the book display where people can sit and look at the books . . . Sometimes they will then purchase one or more of the books, but even if they don't, they have usually found a suggestion of at least one product they will buy before leaving . . .
>
> Any time we sell a book, we know that it will help to generate sales of other items within our stores.

In 1980, more than $50 million was spent for books in health food stores. Nutri-Books, the largest distributor, stocks more than 2,500 books, most of which promote questionable ideas and products. According to its March 1981 catalogue, "the single most important book of the year" is probably *Dr. Atkins' Nutrition Breakthrough,* by Robert C. Atkins, M.D., author of *Dr. Atkins' Diet Revolution* and *Dr. Atkins' Superenergy Diet.*

Dr. Atkins, who practices in New York City, specializes in internal medicine with emphasis on nutrition. According to Attorney Herman Glaser, four lawsuits have been filed against Atkins since 1973 by plaintiffs who believe that they became ill as a result of following the dietary therapy prescribed by Atkins in his first book and in private consultations. Three of the cases were settled out-of-court in favor of the plaintiffs and Atkins successfully defended one case. At a recent hearing where he testified in defense of an RNA product manufacturer, Atkins admitted that he is not certified by the American Board of Internal Medicine because he failed the oral examination and decided not to take it again. (This is a test of the ability to examine patients and make appropriate treatment plans.) But, according to Nutri-Books, Atkins' latest book will have the country "thinking vitamins":

> Dr. Atkins' excellent nationwide reputation and the intensive TV promotion behind the book will send thousands of *totally new customers* into health food stores everywhere.
>
> In *Nutrition Breakthrough* Dr. Atkins, an M.D., is saying just what you've been telling your customers for years— THAT POOR NUTRITION CAUSES MANY DISEASES— THAT GOOD NUTRITION CAN PREVENT AND CURE THOSE DISEASES. Dr. Atkins says that the key is vitamins, minerals and mega-vitamins, AND HE TELLS HIS READERS TO BUY THEM FROM YOU!!!

The book is subtitled *How to Treat Your Medical Condition Without Drugs.* According to an ad by the publisher, Atkins' nutritional system "is not only *safer* but *more effective* than drug oriented treatments, in a wide variety of physical and emotional ailments—everything from headache, depression, anxiety and alcoholism to more serious illnesses such as arthritis, diabetes, heart disease and cancer." The book, a "Main Selection" of Rodale Press's Organic Gardening and Prevention book clubs, also promotes laetrile and "vitamin B_{15}."

Radiance Products Company, a food supplement manufacturer, has recorded a series of "educational nutrition talks" with Dr.

Atkins. "Following release of our first record, on the B-Complex vitamins, our sales of individual B vitamins and B-Complex formulas increased 28%," an ad in *Health Foods Business* reported. Motion pictures of Atkins, which play in a showcase projector, are also available for in-store use.

Syndicate Magazines, "The Total Resource Company," provides health and natural food management with "the only total marketing effort committed to product movement." Larchmont books, one of its divisions, advertises to retailers that they "no longer need to prescribe." Why not? Its 6-book *Preventive Health Library* is "designed to answer many of your customers' questions about the importance of the vitamins you sell." Larchmont also publishes 20 other low-priced paperbacks, including such titles as *Megavitamin Therapy, Minerals: Kill or Cure?* and *The Compleat Herbal.* Most of these books, which contain questionable nutritional ideas, are edited by Ruth Adams (a former editor of *Prevention* Magazine) and Frank Murray, editor of *Health Foods Retailing,* the "official magazine" of the National Nutritional Foods Association.

Syndicate Magazines also publishes *Better Nutrition* and *Today's Living,* monthly magazines that are sold to health food stores for free distribution to customers. Their combined circulation is one million. Typical of health food publications, many of their articles contain claims which would be illegal to make on product labels. Articles occasionally suggest that readers write letters to FDA officials or Congressmen to protest against FDA regulation of supplement sales.

Other Promotional Activities

Many retailers appear on local radio or TV shows where it is legally safe to give advice as long as specific products are not recommended. "Getting on a talk show is not difficult," says an article in *Health Foods Business,* entitled *From Store to Star.* "Nutrition is a popular and controversial subject these days, and you, a health food store owner, are—by definition—an expert on the subject . . . Chances are good that a station in your area would like to do a talk show on the subject, particularly if the guest is an area businessperson."

Viewpoint on Nutrition, a talk show now broadcast free-of-charge by 45 radio and TV stations, was begun in 1970 by the National Nutritional Foods Association. The program's guests are usually food faddists, and its conversations invariably lead to recommendations for "natural" foods and food supplements. Its host is Arnold Pike, D.C., who until recently was NNFA's public information director. In 1981, Pike became director of communications and industry relations for Donsbach University (described later in this chapter), which also assumed sponsorship of the show. On the programs we have watched, Pike was introduced as "Dr. Arnold Pike" and not identified as a chiropractor. Nor were his employment by NNFA or Donsbach University revealed.

Some retailers publish newsletters and many give lectures in their own communities. One has even formed a "separate" educational society which imports guest speakers for public appearances, but most who sponsor prominent guests do so directly. A recent article in *Health Foods Retailing* describes the selling power of prominent lecturers. According to a Nebraska health food store owner, "When Dale Alexander explained the nutritional benefits of cod liver oil, we sold 75 cases of it. I tell you, cod liver oil was going like flowing water." (Alexander claims that cod liver oil reduces the pain of arthritis by lubricating people's joints!)

Prior to the lecture, the store sold one bottle of cod liver oil every few weeks. Now, reports the owner, it sells one or two cases each week. Over 500 hardcover copies of Alexander's books, at $8.95 apiece, were purchased shortly after the lecture. This particular store holds its lectures in a 500-seat auditorium located near the store. Although total costs, including fees, travel expenses and advertising, range from $2,000 to $4,000 per lecturer, the events are profitable both immediately and in the long run.

In *Natural Foods Merchandiser*, a Florida retailer describes how a restaurant can help to "create customers that otherwise would never come into a health food store." The first step is to attract customers by offering low-priced salads and sandwiches. Inside, a large sign near the dining area announces in-store health lectures by a local osteopath who also appears on a daily 5-minute radio show sponsored by the store. Prominent lecturers are imported from time-to-time, and the store also sponsors radio programs by Carlton Fredericks. Vitamin manufacturers who help finance the radio programs are also plugged during the programs.

For $19.95 a month, retailers can subscribe to "Jean's Column Service," a weekly series of health and nutrition advice columns written by Jean Glowka, a former retailer from Rockport, Texas. The columns, *Healthful Hints: Most-Often-Asked Questions on Nutrition*, are set up for publication under the storekeeper's own name with reader questions referred to the store address.

"Newspapers are more than happy to run these without charge," says an article in *Health Foods Business*. "Although the columns subtly promote natural foods and supplements, they are written in language as objective as possible. Like everyone in the industry . . . Glowka must be careful in her wording so that she cannot be misconstrued as prescribing." Each column ends with a disclaimer:

> The above material should not be construed as making claims, endorsements or criticisms. This is merely a relating of facts taken from research done by a number of nutritionists, doctors, scientists, and the author's own experiences.

According to *Health Foods Business*, the quoted experts include Adelle Davis, Linus Pauling, Linda Clark and Roger Williams.

"I never advise anyone to do anything or take anything," says Ms. Glowka. "The disclaimer at the end of the paragraph is very important. It's there to keep me and my subscribers out of hot water with the FDA." As of December 1979, the column was appearing in 30 newspapers and magazines, 20 of them under the sponsorship of retailers.

Oral Claims

Although industry leaders have devised "safe" ways to convey advice "indirectly," retailers actually risk little by making direct oral claims in the relative privacy of a store. Government enforcement efforts, which are quite limited, are directed primarily against manufacturers and distributors of a small number of the more notorious quack remedies such as laetrile. Retailers are generally quite willing to give advice about supplements to their customers.

A striking example of this willingness was reported recently by Sheldon S. Stoffer, M.D., and three associates who operate the Northland Thyroid Laboratory in Southfield, Michigan:

> We surveyed 10 health food distributors by having some of our employees seek out the supervisor or "nutritionist" of each establishment. Our investigators mentioned that their physician was treating them with thyroid hormone because they had a goiter and asked them if they had any products that would help. All 10 advised that they had such useful products. Two advised stopping treatment with thyroid hormone, six advised kelp, two advised iodine tablets, two advised a raw gland preparation containing thyroid, parathyroid, pituitary and adrenal gland extracts, and one advised a raw thyroid preparation . . . Other remedies included turnip tops,

parsnips, parsley, malt tablets, vitamins and mineral supplements. The cost of these preparations per establishment varied from less than $1 to $50.

A few years ago, Eric Faucher, a *National Enquirer* reporter, visited 16 health food stores in major American cities complaining of afternoon fever, weight loss, insomnia and fatigue—symptoms which could indicate a serious disease such as cancer. Only one salesperson told him to see a doctor. The rest prescribed various supplements for such diagnoses as "high blood pressure," "imbalance of energy" and "hypoglycemia." "One salesgirl was stumped by my symptoms," Faucher reported, "so she called up her mother (the store owner) who prescribed vitamin E without ever seeing me!"

Julian DeVries, 76-year-old medical editor of the *Arizona Republic*, recently visited a health food store complaining of weight loss, loss of appetite, insomnia, leg cramps at night and psoriasis (a skin disorder). "Two young clerks sold me an assortment of vitamins for $124.34 that, according to a doctor, easily could have worsened the conditions I told them I had," DeVries reported. Instead of being referred to a physician for *diagnosis* of his possibly serious symptoms, he was sold the following:

1. Megadoses of vitamins B, A and E.
2. A product containing ginseng and an adrenal substance.
3. Digestive enzyme tablets.
4. An iron-and-molasses compound.
5. Tryptophane tablets.
6. A skin cream containing vitamin E and PABA.
7. A book that suggests a nutritional cure for almost every ailment known to man.

Promotion of Herbs

In 1980, health food store patrons spent an estimated $87 million for capsules, tablets and bulk herbs and another $80 million for herbal teas. Although many of these products are being bought for their flavor, it is obvious that many are also being bought for their supposedly medicinal qualities. Paul Goss, proprietor of New Earth Health Foods in Compton, California, suggests that "herbs are a lot cheaper than vitamins . . . and people figure they can keep up their health by taking herbs instead."

E. Paul Larsen, president of Nature's Herbs, Inc., reports that in some parts of the country, "natural" food stores are selling more herbs than vitamins. In an article entitled *Look Out Vitamins, Here Comes Herbs,* he states:

I believe Mother Earth provides a natural herbal "remedy" for every ailment that has ever beset man to help the body help itself. There is no one thing that really "cures" the body. We can only prepare the body and feed it so that it can heal itself.

But according to Peter Dorfman, when he was assistant editor of *Health Foods Business:*

It is generally considered unnecessary and unwise to label herbs as to their uses and medicinal values . . . If an herb is presented as having therapeutic potentials beyond its nutritional value, FDA officials regard it as a drug . . . The retailer who discusses herb products with his customers in terms of their pharmacological uses risks seizure of the products and even criminal charges of prescribing without a license.

We wish this were so. Although Mr. Dorfman stated the law correctly, it is very unlikely to be enforced unless a customer dies as a direct result of poor advice.

Herbs are being promoted—even inside of some stores—by a few traveling lecturers sponsored by herb manufacturers. But most of the promotion is through literature—pamphlets, magazines and books ranging in quality from cheaply printed flyers to elaborately produced studies in fine bindings with attractive art work. Potential customers are rarely told that some herbs are dangerous.

"Practically all of these writings recommend large numbers of herbs for treatment based on hearsay, folklore and tradition," says Varro E. Tyler, Ph.D., dean of Purdue University's schools of pharmacy, nursing and health sciences. "The only criterion which seems to be avoided in these publications is scientific evidence." Dr. Tyler, author of a textbook on plant medicine who is also compiling an authoritative guide to herbs, is horrified at the extent of the claims:

Some writings are so comprehensive and indiscriminate that they seem to recommend everything for anything . . . Even deadly poisonous herbs are sometimes recommended on the basis of some outdated report or a misunderstanding of the facts. Particularly insidious is the myth that there is something almost magical about herbal drugs which prevents them, in their natural state, from harming people.

The most popular magazine promoting herbs is probably *The Herbalist New Health*. Its regular features include testimonials from readers, an "herb of the month," health tips from movie stars and *The Herbalist Mailbox*, which gives "no prescriptive advice" but discusses "historical health building uses of herbs." The magazine also includes many articles that promote a wide variety of food supplements. Most of its ads—including those for laetrile—appear without health claims. However, ads for New Body Products' herbal formulas "RH" and "SH" suggest that they "clean toxins that, because of wrongful diets, build up on nerve endings and result in frustration, sluggish brain, lack of energy and the like," and that they may relieve 42 other problems including acne, high blood pressure, fever, cancer, smoking, lockjaw and "ringworms." (The word "ringworms" does not exist. Perhaps the ad-writer thinks that ringworm is caused by worms. It is caused by a fungus.)

Herbs are also sold person-to-person. The largest company in this field appears to be Nature's Sunshine Products, a division of Amtec Industries, located in Spanish Fork, Utah. Organized like the vitamin companies discussed in Chapter 3, Nature's Sunshine claims to have over 82,000 distributors worldwide and a 1980 sales figure of $14.4 million. A distributor's kit is available to anyone who pays $10 and signs a distributor agreement form acknowledging that "NATURE'S SUNSHINE PRODUCTS are not intended for and are not to be sold as a cure, ameliorant or palliative for any disease or ailment, and that such products are sold solely and only for nutritional purposes."

The kit we obtained does not tell the distributor what "nutritional" value these products are supposed to have. Included, however, are two 2-page flyers which list hundreds of "historical uses of herbs" for the treatment of diseases. One flyer lists individual herbs by name and the other lists the company's herbal products by code letters. The *Distributor Manual* suggests that friends, acquaintances and neighbors be invited to "Herbal Hours in which the traditional usages of herbs, vitamins and other foods or food supplements are discussed . . . It is not a sales meeting. Therefore no Nature's Sunshine Products should be displayed, and no product orders should be taken. An Herbal Hour is an education meeting!" (Sales should be made at another time.)

The manual reminds distributors not to "diagnose," "prescribe," or "make drug claims." It also contains a passage, written by attorney Kirkpatrick W. Dilling, explaining how to avoid trouble with federal drug laws while selling herbs. (Dilling, who has special expertise in defending cases involving questionable health methods, is also attorney for the National Health Federation, a group described in Chapter 10 of this book.) Nature's Sunshine is willing to pay up to $2,000 each to defend distributors accused of diagnosing or prescribing.

Products "for Athletes"

Increasing public interest in fitness has boosted sales of products which are claimed to increase vigor and athletic performance. Chief among them are protein supplements in the form of powders, liquids, tablets and food bars. The health food industry would have us believe that protein plays a special role in the nutrition of athletes or active people. An ad for *Joe Weider's Super Protein Drink* ("The Muscle Drink"), for example, promises:

> . . . to blast giant protein power to your muscles, creating energy, stamina, and building faster muscular gains! . . . to help pack on muscles . . . create energy . . . stamina . . . the space age way for tougher and more enduring workouts.

The scientific facts are otherwise:

1. Proteins are not absorbed as such by the body. Digestion breaks them down to amino acids which are absorbed and become part of the metabolic pool.
2. Amino acids are needed to build or maintain muscles, but muscle-building is not *caused* by eating extra protein. It is stimulated by increased muscular work.
3. Energy, vigor and endurance are related to caloric intake and the availability of adequate energy. Protein is the least efficient source of calories. Athletes will perform better if their extra energy needs are satisfied by extra carbohydrates taken several days before an event takes place.
4. Once basic needs have been met, there is no need for extra protein beyond the Recommended Dietary Allowance. The *small* additional amount needed during intense training is easily obtainable from a balanced diet.

Bee pollen tablets and wheat germ oil are also alleged to improve athletic performance. But neither one contains any nutrients that cannot be supplied less expensively in a balanced diet.

"Nutrition Consultants"

People who sell food supplements typically acquire their knowledge of nutrition by reading popular "nutrition" books and magazines, attending seminars sponsored by supplement manufacturers and distributors, and possibly self-experimentation.

Industry leaders, anxious to upgrade their image, have been devising ways for their salespeople to acquire "credentials."

The most active individual working in this direction is probably Kurt Donsbach, a former health food store operator who was prosecuted 10 years ago for practicing medicine without a license (see Chapter 10). His many projects include Donsbach University (which awards mail-order diplomas in nutrition); the International Academy of Nutrition Consultants (which *anyone* can join for $12); a journal which discusses nutrition topics and carries ads for questionable health products; the International Institute of Natural Health Sciences (which sells publications and provides computerized analysis of "The Nutrient Deficiency Test," a 266-item dietary questionnaire developed by Donsbach); and Health Education Products (a firm that sells publications and food supplement products). According to a Nutri-Books catalogue, *Dr. Donsbach's Nutritional Tape Cassettes,* intended for sale through health food stores, are "like having Dr. Donsbach as your personal physician right in your own home. Each . . . gives pertinent information and direction to aid in diagnosis and remedial action."

Another school that issues mail-order diplomas is Bernadean University, of Van Nuys, California, part of the Church of Universology. The prospectus of its College of Health Sciences offers a 3-credit course in basic nutrition, resulting in a certificate as a "Nutritionist," for $120. A "Cancer Reseacher" certificate can be obtained after a 2-credit-hour course costing $80. Holders of a bachelor's degree can obtain a master's degree if they "write a thesis or take some short course with the school." A doctoral degree ("Ph.D." or "Sc.D.") can then be obtained by taking 36 credit hours (@ $40 per credit) or writing an "equivalent" thesis. "Doctoral" degrees in acupuncture, reflexology, iridology, naturopathy and homeopathy are also available. Richard Passwater, "Ph.D.," is Bernadean's best known graduate. Any student who satisfactorily completes a course may apply for designation as a "school mentor" who can tutor new students. Mentors are also referred to as "Adjunct Professors."

Before moving to California, Bernadean University operated in the state of Nevada. But according to Merlin D. Anderson, Administrator of the Nevada Commission on Postsecondary Education, it was never approved or accredited to offer any courses or degrees. "A Bernadean University degree represents nothing more than a piece of paper," he said recently.

Responding to an inquiry from Dr. Victor Herbert, Robert Welty, consultant to California's Office of Postsecondary Education, wrote that "Bernadean University is operating outside the law in California." Although it has a certificate of incorporation, "that certificate gives them no authorization whatsoever to operate a school or to issue degrees." A few months later, California authorities ordered Bernadean to cease operating.

Another organization, the American Nutrition Consultants Association (ANCA) is open to "anyone interested in the fields of nutritional science and nutritional consultation, and in developing, perfecting and updating one's scope of nutritional knowledge." The only requirements for membership appear to be payment of $25 and completion of an application form which asks for one's name, address, telephone number, gender, age (optional), and professional activities (also optional). Members receive a certificate suitable for framing and *Lifelines*, the monthly ANCA newsletter. The ANCA catalogue defines a "nutrition consultant" as:

> one who is trained in the science of dietetics and nutrition for the purpose of providing information to the public as a consultant in the matters of achieving proper dietary regimes for maintaining a state of optimal health. The profession is often practiced in conjunction with the distribution of health foods and food supplements.

ANCA's president, James D. Flaherty, Ph.D., is also administrator and sole faculty member for a course in nutrition consultation sponsored by his organization. According to him, "The world is waiting for people knowledgeable in nutrition for the purpose of maintaining a state of optimal health . . . These people have the opportunity of becoming a part of the biggest boon to humanity since time began." His 48-lesson course, which costs $100 and must be completed within six months, is based on books written by Kurt Donsbach and himself. Students who finish the course with a "C" average or better are given diplomas, while those who complete it with lower grades are given a "certificate of completion." Flaherty's doctoral degree in nutrition is from Union University, an unaccredited school where Donsbach was affiliated before opening his own school.

The ANCA brochure suggests that "every normal, healthy man, woman and child should seek the advice of a nutritionist for evaluation of his/her nutritional needs." So should people involved in active sports, children, teenagers, pregnant women, persons suffering from chronic diseases, individuals on medication, people with weight problems, people over 60 and people in job or life-related stress situations. (Do you know anyone not covered by this list?)

A recent article in *Health Foods Business* suggests that health food stores should work toward achieving professional status. "It's likely that the health food store of the future will have a certified nutritionist on its staff—the equivalent of a pharmacist in a drug store," the article states. "Health food store owners—and the whole industry—should begin thinking about how such a system of accreditation from a recognized and respected institution might work."

The National Nutritional Foods Association is thinking along these lines. Early in 1981, a membership mailing promised that its annual convention would offer a "nutrition counseling" seminar certified by the College of Continuing Education, University of Southern California (USC), for "four hours of continuing education contact under qualified academic instruction" sponsored by NNFA. (The instructor was to have been a foreign-trained physician who is not licensed to practice medicine in the United States.) Participants in the $15 seminar were to receive certificates to display in their stores. According to a USC official, however, NNFA's announcement was both inaccurate and premature. "Plans for a course in *basic nutrition concepts* were merely under *discussion* and were never finalized. After the announcement was made, and the person at NNFA who was communicating with us was replaced, further discussions were terminated by mutual agreement."

Arthritis Quackery

There is hardly a food item which has not been promoted at one time or another as a "cure" for arthritis. Medical research has found only one form of arthritis (gout) whose symptoms are partially related to the type of food eaten. Yet myths persist that dietary factors can cause or cure other arthritic conditions.

Diets based on raw foods, foods without chemical additives and other supposedly "natural" nutrition items are being hustled by the health food industry. So are misleading books which, unfortunately, have been best sellers. "Natural" faddists overlook the fact that prehistoric man—who certainly ate no additives—also suffered from arthritis. This fact has been documented by bone studies.

One of the most recent "natural" products promoted for arthritis is an extract from the green-lipped mussel, a shellfish found only in the waters off New Zealand. Since no scientific evidence of this product's safety or effectiveness has been submitted to the FDA, the FDA has banned its importation into the U.S.

"Diagnostic Methods"

The health food industry has not been content to merely treat the full range of illnesses with nutritional methods. It has also developed its own methods of "diagnosis." The latest rage is hair analysis. Health food stores, nutrition consultants, chiropractors and some other licensed practitioners are employing this procedure, and some companies even offer the test by mail to readers of health food magazines. Dr. Atkins even offers to arrange a test for readers of his latest book.

To obtain the test, customers are instructed to furnish a sample of hair, usually from the back of the neck, which is sent to a laboratory for analysis. The customer and/or the referring source then get back a computerized printout that supposedly indicates deficiencies or excesses of minerals. Some also report supposed deficiencies of vitamins. One mail-order laboratory recently recommended that a man in apparently good physical health take a total of 34 doses of 17 different supplement products daily. Included were "vitamin B_{15}" and 40,000 units of vitamin A (a potentially toxic dosage).

An article in *Let's Live* magazine suggests that "if you or anyone in your family has a history of cancer, diabetes, hypertension, or any one of dozens of other debilitating diseases, you and your family need to have your hair analyzed." The article then reports a study of a church group in which "not a single patient has a completely normal distribution of minerals" and "35 percent of this population had toxic levels of heavy minerals." (Does the fear-magic pitch sound familiar?)

Do you suffer from "chronic health problems like fatigue, depression or headaches"? According to ads in *Let's Live* and *Prevention*, "heavy metal accumulations in your body may be the cause." For only $20 plus a sample of your hair, you can receive a report which "could suggest simple lifestyle and dietary changes which may aid in relief from fatigue, chronic anxiety, and pains you never thought would go away."

Bertram A. Spilker, M.D., Ph.D., a government consultant, recently sent six samples of hair from each of three healthy young adults to three different laboratories for analysis. Included were duplicate samples from each individual—one from each side of the back of the head. The reported results varied not only from lab to lab, but also from sample to sample of the same individual. But even if testing were to yield consistent results, the fact is that *the state of the body's health may be completely unrelated to the chemical composition of the hair*. Hair analysis may have some limited usefulness in the diagnosis of lead, cadmium, arsenic or mercury poisoning, but using it as a routine test is a waste of money. Hair analysis can *not* diagnose vitamin deficiency because there are no vitamins in hair except at the root (below the surface of the skin). Nor can it diagnose mineral deficiency because lower limits for "normal" values of minerals in hair have not been established.

The mineral composition of hair can be affected by a person's age, natural hair color, and rate of hair growth—as well as by the use of hair dyes, bleaches and shampoos. Some dandruff shampoos contain zinc or selenium, and some hair dyes contain lead. When these products are used, some laboratories will report that the user is being "poisoned"! Worse yet, some then recommend "treatment" with ETDA, a drug that can destroy the kidneys.

Some practitioners are also using computer analysis of diet as a diagnostic test. This may seem modern and scientific, but almost all of these computers are programmed to suggest unnecessary food supplements.

A Criminal Prosecution

Hair analysis was involved in a case prosecuted in 1980 by the Los Angeles City Attorney's Office. According to the official press release, Benjamin Colimore and his wife, Sarah, owners of a health food store, would take hair samples from customers in order to diagnose and treat various conditions. The Colimores were also co-hosts of a weekly radio talk show on nutrition, but the case was not related to statements made on their show.

Prosecution was initiated after a customer complained that the Colimores had said she had a bad heart valve and was suffering from abscesses of the pancreas, arsenic in her system, and benign growths of the liver, intestine and stomach—all based on analysis of her hair. Two substances were prescribed, an "herbal tea" which turned out to be only milk sugar, and "Arsenicum," another milk sugar product that contained traces of arsenic.

Another sample of hair was taken when the customer returned to the store five weeks later. She was told that the earlier conditions were gone, but that she now had lead in her stomach. A government investigator received similiar diagnosis and treatment. After pleading "no contest" to one count of practicing medicine without a license, the Colimores were fined $2,000, given a 60-day suspended jail sentence and placed on probation for two years.

Nutrition Roulette

The health food industry has a huge number of "treatment" methods. Thousands of food supplement products are being produced by hundreds of manufacturers, and a wide variety of foods are also being promoted for their supposedly special health-giving properties. The overall industry philosophy seems to be that anything is worth trying for anything and that "more is better" when it comes to dosage. Its salespeople may not understand biochemistry, but they do understand how to sell.

The degree of danger in following advice from a popular publication, a health food store clerk or a "nutrition consultant," varies with the degree of customer belief and the presence or absence of significant illness. Reliance upon an unproven method can endanger your health or your life in addition to your pocketbook. But it is clear that on a person-to-person basis, anyone can get away with recommending almost any type of "treatment" for almost any health problem.

Chapter 5

"Passive" Greed?

Although pharmacy is a science, and although pharmacists are scientifically trained, drugstores actually sell more vitamins than do health food stores. *Health Foods Business* estimates that the sale of supplements in health food stores amounted to $557 million in 1980. But surveys reported by drug trade publications suggest that pharmacies sold considerably more.

Pharmacy schools correctly teach their students that people who eat a balanced diet rarely need supplements. But after they graduate, pharmacists are seldom reminded of this fact. The subject of vitamin overuse is rarely mentioned in their scientific journals, and their trade publications talk only about vitamin promotion. A 1978 article in *Drug Topics*, for example, tells pharmacists how to take advantage of the growing public interest in food supplements:

> One way to stay ahead of consumer buying patterns is to keep tabs on what customers are reading—health food magazines, nutrition articles in women's magazines or any of the more popular paperback vitamin books . . . By keeping track of what is happening in the health food store trade right now, you can get the jump on what might be happening in drugstore vitamin sales six months from now . . .
>
> A trend that underscores the need for a complete vitamin line is the continuing segmentation of the market into target categories. First came special formulations for women containing iron; now there are special vitamins for men containing zinc (said to aid prostate problems). Today there are vitamins tailored for different age groups, stress formulas for the anxious, and energy compounds for the athletes—especially joggers. Just now appearing on the shelves are vitamins aimed specifically at strengthening the hair, and another new product advertises itself as a beauty formula . . .
>
> "The vitamin business is not unlike the fashion industry," says one expert. "What sells depends upon what is in vogue." The difference is that while manufacturers and designers set

48

the styles in fashions, in vitamins it's the customers with the latest scientific findings in hand who determine sales trends.

Accompanying the *Drug Topics* article is a list of "popular claims for top-selling dietary supplements," including lecithin ("flushes cholesterol out of the bloodstream"), zinc ("said to retard senility"), dolomite ("calming effect on nerves"), selenium ("possibly aiding in the prevention of cancer and heart disease"), and B_{15} or pangamic acid ("superenergy panacea").

Do you think these are the "latest scientific findings"? The article's author apparently does not:

> This list is not a medical endorsement of claims, but simply a guide to what customers believe about the food supplements they purchase. Dietary supplements are considered foods by the Food and Drug Administration, and as such, are generally not subject to the premarket approval requirements for safety and efficacy that drugs are. Vitamin and mineral supplements are not permitted to carry drug labeling claims relative to the treatment of disease.

(Translation: *Since it is illegal to lie on a product label, the health food industry must rely on other channels of communication to mislead its customers.*)

Do you think it is ethical for pharmacists to profit from the confusion of their customers? According to Carl Short, marketing director for P. Leiner & Sons, a private label manufacturer, "The smart merchandiser is going to stock what people want." Tom Nickel, vitamin marketing for Rexall Drug Company, advises pharmacists to convey the idea that their drugstore has a "total" vitamin department so that the customer doesn't have to shop elsewhere. He also suggests that merchandising health-related paperbacks and magazines next to the vitamin section is a good technique. (The ones which promote supplements, of course.)

William H. Lee believes "There's an entire world out there that no one told us about in pharmacy school." (Why do you suppose they aren't told?) Described in *American Druggist* as a pharmacist who works as a consultant and specializes in the health food field, Lee states:

> Even if you do not carry health-related paperbacks as a rule, you must put in and sell health-related titles. They will be your best salesmen. People will read about the use of various vitamins and minerals. You as a pharmacist may not be able to

recommend a certain combination for a certain condition. The law forbids you to do it. But if a person chooses to follow a path because he believes it will do him some good, then he has a right to buy and try what he wishes.

(Translation: *You can't lie, so let the books lie for you.*)

Looking into the future, Lee sees pharmacists using desktop computers to prescribe supplements by analyzing questionnaires filled out by customers. Do you think the computers he envisions would ever tell anyone not to buy supplements?

Advertising Tactics

Health food industry propaganda is not the only reason why vitamin sales are booming.* Advertising by so-called "ethical" manufacturers—now at the level of $60 million a year—is also a major factor. In the past, much of this advertising was done to persuade drugstores to stock their brands. Today, however, there is greater emphasis on advertising to the general public. For example:

• E. R. Squibb & Sons advertises that *Theragran* was selected by the U.S. Olympic Team. Does that sound impressive? Two facts are not mentioned in the ads, however. One is that world-class athletes are among the people *least* likely to need supplements. The other is that Olympic endorsements are *purchased!* In Theragran's case, the price was $500,000.

Another Squibb ad has featured tennis star Billie Jean King recommending *Theragran* because "you can never do enough for yourself." It is amusing to recall the celebrated "Battle of the Sexes" years ago when Mrs. King trounced her male opponent, Bobby Riggs, despite his intake of vitamin pills by the fistful. Do you suppose a single *Theragran* is more powerful than fistfuls of other pills? Or could Riggs have been weakened by vitamin overdosage?

• The J. B. Williams Company has a cleverly-worded ad: "IF YOU HAVE IRON POOR BLOOD ALL THE VITAMINS IN THE

---

*When we speak of the "health food industry," we refer mostly to promoters who greatly exaggerate the value of nutrients or use blatant scare tactics associated with a basic rejection of scientific facts. "Ethical" manufacturers who promote "nutritional insurance" with more subtle scare tactics may be equally guilty of profiteering, although most of their other thinking is rooted in science. Some distinction should also be made between owner-operated and chain-operated drugstores. The latter are far more likely to be unprincipled in their vitamin promotions.

WORLD WON'T HELP. Iron poor blood is the most widespread nutritional ailment in America today. And taking vitamins won't help, because vitamins don't contain iron. What you need is Geritol, every day . . ."

We beg to differ. The ad doesn't say how you are supposed to know whether you have iron-poor blood (anemia). But if you really have it, what you need is not *Geritol* but medical supervision. If your anemia happens to be caused by internal bleeding—by a curable cancer in its early stages, for example—what you need is a *diagnosis* before it is too late. Conversely, if you take iron and don't need it, you can develop iron overload disease which can damage your pancreas, liver and heart.

If you become anemic as a result of poor nutrition, you should develop better eating habits. Sufficient dietary iron can be obtained by cooking in a "Dutch oven" or any iron pot or by eating iron-rich foods such as soy beans, liver, veal muscle or almost any other meat. Women who have excessively heavy menstrual periods may need to take iron supplements, but this should be done under the supervision of a physician who first determines the presence of iron-deficiency anemia by using a blood test. Iron-containing products should be handled with some caution. There are about 2,000 cases of iron poisoning each year in the United States, mainly in children who ingest the medicinal supplements of their parents.

• Hudson Pharmaceuticals uses radio commercials geared toward "seasonal trends" in vitamin sales. In January/February 1980, vitamins were suggested to counter the supposed effects of stress. Fun and fitness were featured in March and April. May/June used a "natural" theme, and September related vitamins to going back to school. In 1981, Hudson began "Nutra-Phone," a daily "educational" message on nutrition and health that can be heard by dialing a telephone number in New York City. Not surprisingly, many of its messages use scare tactics to promote the sale of unnecessary supplements.

• Hoffmann-La Roche, Inc., *which produces most of the bulk nutrients repackaged by other vitamin manufacturers*, advertises heavily to both the public and the medical profession. The company maintains a Vitamin Nutrition Information Service which distributes reports that quote scientific literature but are heavily biased toward vitamin supplementation—exaggerating the need and minimizing the risks by omitting adverse facts.

When a manufacturer plans a major advertising campaign, it will be publicized first in drug trade publications so that druggists can stock up on the products promoted.

Ethical Questions

Virtually all drugstores carry a large assortment of vitamin products, including some "natural" ones. While almost all chain stores promote them vigorously, most individually owned ones do not. Some pharmacies use deceptive tactics (like placing vitamin C products among cold remedies or vitamin A with eye care products), while others display their vitamins inconspicuously.

If asked point blank, most pharmacists will admit that few of their customers need supplements and that megadoses of vitamins should be taken only under medical supervision. Why, then, do they stock and sell them willingly? Many pharmacists claim that if they try to discourage vitamin purchases, most customers will get angry and shop elsewhere. Do you think this is true? (Would these pharmacists be willing to post signs stating: "You don't need supplements, but if you've been talked into them, we'll be happy to sell them to you."?) Or do you think the bottom line is money? According to an article in Drug Topics, "the vitamin category is one of the drugstore's top money-makers. For the space it requires, nothing equals the vitamin section for fast turnover (typically 5-7 times a year) and large profits."

In our opinion, *pharmacists have as much of an ethical duty to discourage unnecessary use of vitamin and mineral supplements as physicians do to advise against unnecessary surgery or medical care.* Do you know of any pharmacists who do so?

Has any pharmacist, pharmacy school professor or professional pharmaceutical organization ever made a *sustained* effort to speak out *publicly* against the fraudulent promotion of unnecessary food supplements? Is there a conspiracy of silence? Is there any reason why the pharmaceutical profession should not make a *determined political effort* to protect Americans from being misled by major pharmaceutical manufacturers as well as the health food industry? Can't pharmacies exist without selling products to people who don't need them?

Chapter 6

Dubious Doctoring

Unlicensed operators are not the only ones advocating unnecessary nutrients or engaging in questionable nutritional practices. Some physicians and dentists, and many chiropractors and naturopaths are also involved.

Physicians quite properly recommend vitamins for very young children until they are eating solid foods which contain enough vitamins. After the age of two, however, it is seldom necessary to continue supplements "just to be sure." In 1980, the Committee on Nutrition of the American Academy of Pediatrics addressed this issue in a lengthy statement which began as follows:

> The last 50 years have witnessed a steadily increasing understanding of the biochemistry of vitamins and trace minerals and their role in human nutrition . . .
>
> As nutritional needs became more clearly defined, essential vitamins and minerals were incorporated into processed formulas with the aim of providing an essentially complete food for infants; specific nutrients likely to be lacking in the diet of older infants and children were used to fortify certain food products, such as infant cereal. Supplemental vitamin and mineral drops or tablets continued to be used, probably to a greater extent than necessary considering the more extensive fortification of food.

The committee's guidelines for supplementation include the following (rewritten in our words):

1. All newborn infants should receive vitamin K to prevent hemorrhagic disease of the newborn. (This is standard medical practice.)
2. Fluoride supplements should be given to infants and children in communities whose water supply is not fluoridated.
3. Children with poor eating habits and those on weight-reduction diets can be given a multivitamin-mineral supplement containing nutrients at not more than RDA levels.

(Improving eating habits is of course preferable to supplementation.)

4. Pregnant teenagers are likely to need supplementary iron and folic acid. (This is also true for pregnant adults.)
5. Children on strict vegetarian diets without adequate animal protein from dairy products or eggs may need supplementation, particularly with vitamin B_{12}.
6. There is no evidence that supplementation is necessary for the properly nourished child. (Properly nourished simply means eating from the four basic food groups each day.)

What about adults? Unfortunately, many physicians prescribe vitamins or "tonics" to adults who complain of fatigue or depression. Although this may pacify some patients, it also reinforces health food industry mythology.

Fad Diagnoses

A small number of physicians—no more than one or two per thousand—are engaged in "nutritional" practices that are rejected as quackery by scientific practitioners. Often they refer to themselves as "holistic," "metabolic," "unorthodox," "alternative" or "nutritional" doctors.

A few years ago, many nervous or tired people were said to have "adrenal insufficiency," a serious glandular disorder which is actually quite rare. The vast majority of these people were not only misdiagnosed, but were also treated with adrenal gland extract, a substance they didn't need and which is potentially harmful.

Today, "hypoglycemia" (low blood sugar) is fashionable as a socially acceptable diagnosis to explain away certain symptoms of neurotic nervousness or fatigue. This condition, which is extremely rare, should be diagnosed only after careful interpretation of a blood sugar test. A diagnosis of functional hypoglycemia should not be considered unless a person on a balanced diet gets symptoms 2-4 hours after eating and also develops blood glucose levels below 45 mg per 100 ml *whenever symptoms occur* during a glucose tolerance test. Low blood sugar levels without symptoms occur commonly in normal individuals fed large amounts of sugar and are therefore of no diagnostic significance. Doctors who are "true believers" in "hypoglycemia" are likely to diagnose it in a large percentage of their patients. Such doctors are also likely to be unscientific or even unscrupulous practitioners. Nutrition is not a belief system; it is a science.

A few physicians claim that millions of people are suffering from "cerebral allergies." Some of these doctors call themselves "clinical ecologists." They speculate that common foods, food additives, cooking gas, perfumes, pesticides and other chemicals can interfere with the body's enzyme systems to cause fatigue, nausea, anxiety, severe depression and even schizophrenia. Treatment, which is usually quite expensive, involves elimination diets, special rooms sealed off from outside air, enzymes taken by mouth and large doses of vitamins and minerals. Because the number of chemicals to which we are exposed in tiny amounts is enormous, and because the symptoms these substances are supposed to cause are prone to come and go by themselves, speculations of this sort are virtually impossible to test. We know, however, that the enzymes prescribed by these practitioners are inactivated by the stomach and intestines, and are usually not absorbed in sufficient quantity to function elsewhere in the body as enzymes.

"Miracle" Drugs

Gerovital H3 (GH3) was developed by Anna Aslan, a Rumanian physician. It is being promoted by the Rumanian National Tourist Office and a few American physicians as an anti-aging substance—"the secret of eternal vigor and youth." Claims have been made that GH3 can prevent or relieve a wide variety of disorders, including arthritis, arteriosclerosis, angina pectoris and other heart conditions, neuritis, deafness, Parkinson's disease, depression, senile psychosis and impotence. It is also claimed to stimulate hair growth, to repigment gray hair, and to tighten and smoothen skin. (The very length of this list should make you suspicious of the claims.) Although many uncontrolled studies describe great benefits from the use of GH3, controlled trials have failed to demonstrate any improvement in elderly patients. One astute observer has remarked that GH3 only seems to work in Rumania.

The main ingredient in GH3 is procaine, a local anesthetic which can cause convulsions and other serious side effects when rapidly absorbed. Such complications are rare, however. Noting that para-aminobenzoic (PABA) acid appears in the urine of people receiving procaine injections, a few American manufacturers have been selling "procaine tablets" containing PABA with false claims similar to those made for GH3.

"Chelation therapy" involves injection of disodium edetate or ETDA into the bloodstream where it supposedly cleans out unwanted mineral deposits from various parts of the body before exiting via the kidneys. A course of treatment consisting of 20-50 injections can cost thousands of dollars. According to its promoters, chelation therapy may be helpful in kidney and heart disease, arthritis, Parkinson's disease, emphysema, multiple sclerosis, gangrene, psoriasis . . . (need we go on?). Chelation therapy can cause death from kidney destruction. Although many people claim that chelation therapy has helped them, such testimony is not evidence that it works. *People who believe in a product may feel better even while it is killing them.*

Procaine PVP, another injectable substance, was developed by Peter T. DeMarco, M.D., and used for the treatment of cancer, heart disease and many other ailments. In 1978, Dr. DeMarco's New Jersey medical license was revoked after a hearing at which it was charged that his neglect of sterile technique resulted in 92 cases of hepatitis. His Pennsylvania license was then revoked also.

Chelation therapy (except for heavy metal poisoning) and treatment with GH3 and procaine PVP do not have FDA approval, and physicians who use these treatments may be operating on the fringes of the law. We suggest that you steer clear of anyone who even recommends these methods.

Megavitamin Therapy

About 30 years ago, a small number of psychiatrists began adding massive doses of nutrients to their treatment of severe mental problems. The original substance used was vitamin B_3 (nicotinic acid or nicotinamide), and the use of enormous vitamin doses was termed "megavitamin therapy." Since that time, the treatment regimen has expanded to include vitamins, minerals, hormones and diets, any of which may be combined with conventional drug therapy and/or electroshock treatments. Today the treatment is called "orthomolecular psychiatry," a term defined as "the treatment of mental disease by the provision of optimal molecular environment for the mind, especially substances normally present in the human body." In practice, the word "optimum" alway seems to mean "more."

Abram Hoffer, M.D., Ph.D., a Canadian psychiatrist who was one of the originators of megavitamin therapy, claims that "orthomolecular psychiatry has already cured, or greatly aided in the recovery of over 30,000 patients who were previously given up as hopeless cases not worth any further effort on the part of a physician or psychiatrist." (We do not believe this claim.) Dr. Hoffer is also president of the New York City-based Huxley Institute for Biosocial Research, parent organization of the American Schizophrenia Association. The institute claims to have 3,000 members and "over 9,000 loyal contributors." It distributes a list of about 140 psychiatrists and other physicians whose scope of practice includes schizophrenia, hypoglycemia, depression, learning and behavioral disorders, alcoholism, allergies, senility and/or "preventive medicine."

One of the more prominent centers for "orthomolecular medicine" is the Brain Bio Center of Princeton, New Jersey. Its $255 fee for an initial visit covers a history ($30) and a consultation with a physician ($60), plus hair analysis ($25) and various other laboratory tests that most psychiatrists would not consider necessary or useful in the diagnosis of mental disorders. Follow up visits at the center cost from $38 to $150, depending on the number of laboratory tests performed. These fees do not include the cost of prescribed vitamins.

A special task force of the American Psychiatric Association has investigated the claims of the megavitamin and orthomolecular therapists. Its report, issued in 1973, concludes:

> This review and critique has carefully examined the literature produced by megavitamin proponents and by those who have attempted to replicate their basic and clinical work. It concludes that . . . the credibility of the megavitamin proponents is low. Their credibility is further diminished by a consistent refusal over the past decade to perform controlled experiments and to report their results in a scientifically acceptable fashion. Under these circumstances this Task Force considers the massive publicity which they promulgate via radio, the lay press and popular books, using catch phrases which are really misnomers like "megavitamin therapy" and "orthomolecular treatment," to be deplorable.

The Research Advisory Committee of the National Institute of Mental Health has reviewed pertinent scientific data through 1979 and agrees that orthomolecular therapy is ineffective and may be harmful. After the U.S. Senate Defense Subcommittee looked into this therapy, it was removed as a covered treatment under the CHAMPUS insurance program for military dependents.

Dubious Dentistry

A number of dentists—led by Hal Huggins, D.D.S., of Colorado Springs, Colorado—have been promoting the notion of "balancing body chemistry." These dentists claim that dietary practices can prevent a wide variety of "degenerative" diseases. Special diets and expensive food supplements are recommended to achieve "balance," and questionable laboratory tests (such as hair analysis) are used with false claims that they can determine the biochemical state of the patient. Supporters of these methods greatly exaggerate and misrepresent what nutrition can do. Their patients acquire false hopes and waste money.

Like all of the health professions, dentistry has individuals who abuse their dental degrees by promoting questionable methods for patients who are hopelessly ill. One such dentist is William D. Kelley who, for many years, operated a clinic and computer laboratory in Grapevine, Texas. Kelley claims that cancer is caused by "inadequate production or utilization of enzymes." His book, *One Answer to Cancer*, claims that cancer can be diagnosed by "simple urinalysis," that it "often can be controlled by diet alone," and that it can "almost always be controlled by proper dosage of enzymes." He claims that his Kelley Malignancy Index is " the most accurate and extensive cancer detection system ever developed." It is supposed to determine "the presence or absence of cancer, the growth rate of the tumor, the location of the tumor mass, prognosis of the treatment, age of the tumor and the regulation of medication for treatment."

After many years of difficulty with various federal and state law enforcement agencies, Kelley lost his Texas dental license and relocated in Winthrop, Washington. In 1976, he formed the Nutritional Academy and began requiring that anyone wishing to consult him must first become, for a $5 fee, an Academy member. According to Cameron Stauth, editor of the *National Journal of the Nutritional Academy:*

> This not only provided an initial membership for the "club," but was also a sensible action legally—in our political framework, anyone who offers "treatment" to the "general public" is vulnerable to intense scrutiny and political pressure by the medico/political authorities . . . By creating an "association" where only members could come for consultation and by refusing to provide "treatment" with drugs, surgery or other forms of "invasive" therapy, Dr. Kelley circumvented the whole problem of "treating the general public."

In 1978, membership in the Academy increased from about 100 to about 5,000, and a network of "counselors" was developed throughout the United States. In 1980, the Academy was renamed the International Health Institute (IHI). Its "nutrition counselors," now called "Certified Metabolic Technicians," promise a "complete progressive health care and metabolic life style program." The much-publicized but futile effort to cure actor Steve McQueen's cancer was conducted under Dr. Kelley's guidance. This "treatment," which included a protein-deficient diet, laetrile and coffee enemas, may even have hastened McQueen's death.

Certification as a Metabolic Technician requires a course which costs $1,400, not including food supplements. Students must personally use the Kelley nutritional program and supervise three others who do so. Kelley's Institute was advertised in the October 1980 issue of *Prevention* magazine. Respondents to the ad received an informational packet plus a letter from their nearest "metabolic technician."

IHI's main objective, as stated in its "Declaration of Purpose," is to "restore, maintain and improve the health of every member and of every citizen of the United States of America." The Institute is prepared to file lawsuits to protect "the basic right of our members to select spokesmen from their number who could be expected to give wisest counsel and advice concerning matters of nutrition, food, natural living, and all aspects of total health." But it "does not, nor will it ever, advocate the violent overthrow of the Government of these United States of America."

Membership in IHI is open to any individual who pays $10 and signs an application asserting that he is not a government agent, that he will never aid a government agency that brings any action against the Institute, that neither he (nor his heirs) will ever sue or bring a criminal charge against the Institute, and that he will never divulge any information about the Institute to any investigator. (Do you think Dr. Kelley is nervous about something?)

Chiropractors

Chiropractic is based upon the belief that most ailments are the result of spinal problems. The "discovery" of chiropractic was announced in 1895 by Daniel David Palmer, a grocer and "magnetic healer" who practiced in Davenport, Iowa. Palmer believed that he had restored the hearing of a partially deaf janitor by "adjusting" a bump on his spine. After further thought, he decided that the basic cause of disease is "nerve interference" caused by misaligned spinal bones which could be adjusted back into place by hand.

Today's 24,000 chiropractors (D.C.s) can be divided into two general groups. "Straight" chiropractors cling strictly to Palmer's basic doctrines. The rest—referred to as "mixers"—acknowledge that factors such as germs and hormones play a role in disease, but they regard mechanical disturbances as the *underlying* cause of lowered resistance to disease. Mixers use dietary methods and various forms of physiotherapy in addition to spinal manipulation.

Chiropractors generally tend to give credibility to the questionable claims of food faddists described elsewhere in this book. Nutrition articles in chiropractic journals almost always exaggerate what nutrients can do. Most of the journals contain many ads for vitamins and other food supplement products, some of which are misbranded. Seminars sponsored by the largest chiropractic organization (American Chiropractic Association) feature speakers like Carlton Fredericks and Emanuel Cheraskin (see Chapter 8). Seminars sponsored by food supplement companies and "chiropractic nutritionists" recommend a variety of highly questionable nutritional methods, including quack cancer remedies.

Although some aspects of scientific nutrition are taught in chiropractic schools, most of the ideas which chiropractors absorb are as unscientific as their own basic theory of disease. Chiropractors who give nutritional advice typically recommend vitamin supplements which we would consider unnecessary. Many of these chiropractors sell the supplements themselves at twice their cost or more. Some chiropractors—probably several hundred—charge *thousands* of dollars for treatment programs which include diagnostic evaluations, vitamins, adjustments and massage during a period of several months.

The following nutritionally-related activities are among those which have been widely advertised to chiropractors during the past few years:

• The International Academy of Chiropractic Nutritionists offers "The Triple Your Income—Nutrition Seminar," a 2-day program "to learn the real dynamic power of a successful nutrition practice—not some superficial scheme." Its methods, "worth millions of dollars in a lifetime of practice," promise to correct such problems as ulcers, prostate problems, colds, impotency, hemorrhoids, depression, kidney stones and bladder stones "in a matter of a few days."

• The Doctors' Seminar on Nutrition, according to its brochure, is taught by "the two most knowledgeable men in nutrition available on the American scene today." One is John Courtney, vice president of Standard Process Laboratories and "the most knowledgeable man in nutritional research today." This company, a division of Vitamin Products Company, Milwaukee, Wisconsin, was founded by the late Royal Lee, a nonpracticing dentist who was described in 1963 by a prominent FDA official as "probably the largest publisher of unreliable and false nutritional information in the world." Brochures for the Doctors' Seminar state that Mr. Courtney "worked closely with Dr. Lee for more than 30 years." Government prosecution of Dr. Lee and his company is detailed in Chapter 10.

The other seminar instructor is Richard Murray, D.C., who "practices more nutrition than any other doctor in America . . . He uses in excess of $200,000 of Standard Process products each year." (Cost of food supplements to the doctor, that is!) The 15-hour course, which costs $175 to attend, is also available on tape. "Nearly a thousand doctors listened to Dr. Murray in seminar during 1978," a brochure states. One of its covered subjects is "successful handling of multiple sclerosis, muscular dystrophy, impotency and mental disorders." Food supplements have no legitimate role in the treatment of these conditions—but no matter. One of Dr. Lee's principles, listed in Standard Process Laboratory's booklet *Applications of Nutritional Principles for the Chiropractic Profession,* is: "A fact need not be 'proved' to be useful."

• Dee Cee Laboratories, a food supplement company that also operates as Nutra-Val Nutritional Services, provides chiropractors with "nutritional questionnaires" for their patients to complete. The forms are then analyzed by a computer which supposedly can "evaluate the nutrients you are presently low in." The form states that it "is not designed for the purpose of diagnosing, prescribing or treatment of disease. Its purpose is to evaluate your nutritional status and to determine if you are consuming the right nutrients in the proper proportions." The computer is programmed to recommend various Dee Cee formulas which can be purchased from the chiropractor (at 2-3 times his cost) or shipped directly from Dee Cee to the patient. The report costs the doctor $10, and its suggested cost to the patient is $20 or $25.

Although ads for the questionnaire suggest that it is "a complete nutritional evaluation," only 4 of its 132 questions even ask about the patient's eating habits. The rest refer to nonspecific symptoms. Some of the symptoms may occur in vitamin deficiency disease or glandular dysfunction, but many of them have nothing whatsoever to do with nutritional status. Nor would we recommend any of Dee Cee's products for the treatment of glandular disorders.

• Linblads, Inc., of Dearborn, Michigan, sponsors many free

seminars to promote chiropractic use of products made by Nutri-Dyn Products, Inc., "the fastest growing nutritional company in the United States." The products include vitamin-mineral mixtures, homeopathic remedies, and "raw gland concentrates," many of which are named after body parts—*Cardiotrophic Concentrate, Mammarytrophic, Nutri-Derm, Prostadyn*, etc. Literature distributed by Linblads claims that its various products are valuable in the treatment of more than 100 serious disorders, including cancer.

In 1976, Robert F. Linblad, Elmer A. Linblad and Linblads, Inc., were convicted and fined a total of $7,000 for marketing a misbranded and unapproved drug. We believe that many of its current products are equally questionable, but the FDA has not brought prosecution.

Linblads has also been promoting "metabolic health seminars" by Harold Manner, Ph.D., the University of Loyola (Chicago) biology professor who achieved notoriety in 1977 by claiming to have cured cancer in mice with injections of laetrile, enzymes and vitamin A. What he actually did was *digest* the tumors by injecting digestive enzymes into them (the equivalent of sticking a red-hot poker into them), but this cannot affect cancer that has spread. Since then Dr. Manner has developed "nutritional" approaches which he claims can help many other serious diseases.

A California chiropractor who uses the "Manner Metabolic Therapy Program" has patients spend six hours a day at his clinic, three days a week for three weeks. In addition to "nutritional detoxification," the program may include chiropractic manipulation, physical therapy, colonic therapy, psychological and nutritional counseling, exercise, relaxation, and preparation of foods and juices. The fee for the three weeks— a mere $2,500—includes all of the above plus food supplements, lab tests and doctor fees. Living expenses and a (required) juicer are extra.

Similar "treatment" is available at the Health and Wellness Center of Bloomington, Minnesota, whose director holds a "Ph.D." from Donsbach University. The Center's brochure, which lists Dr. Manner as its "Chief Consultant for the Metabolic Program for Cancer," states that more than 100 locations now offer his recommended program.

• The New Breed Nutrition Club, of Belen, New Mexico, chapter 8364 of the Basic Bible Club of America, is "dedicated to research and education concerning NUTRITION and the PHILOSOPHY OF OPTIMAL HEALTH." Its letterhead lists 24 promoters of questionable "nutrition" practices, including H. Ray Evers,

M.D. (chelation therapist), Richard Passwater (promoter of selenium and "B_{15}"), Benjamin Frank, M.D. (now deceased, whose
book claims that eating sardines can make you look younger),
Ernesto Contreras, M.D. (world's leading dispenser of laetrile),
and three people convicted of laetrile-related crimes. Club literature stresses that its "systems and programs are never intended to
diagnose, treat, ameliorate or cure any disease or condition. They
are designed to be oriented towards the nutritional, biochemical,
metabolic and physiologic aspects of the human body."

Membership in the New Breed Nutrition Club is open to anyone
free-of-charge. Professional membership requires merely a signed
statement that one is a "nutrition or health professional in good
standing in your community." Laypersons may join by filling out,
signing and forwarding (with a $35 check) a "Nutriscope Calcula-
tor," a booklet containing 570 questions and spaces for a one-week
diary of food intake, symptoms, and test of urine and saliva acid-
ity. The booklet's last page is a membership agreement (required
for processing) acknowledging that the prospective club member
"is participating in an ongoing research project," is seeking only
"nutritional assistance . . . not medical or diagnostic advice," and
is not "an agent for federal, state or local agencies on a mission of
entrapment or investigation."

Why the disclaimers? Scoring of the booklet is done by Alan H.
Nittler, M.D., club founder and executive director, who sends
"nutritional" recommedations to the referring health professional. Presumably, Dr. Nittler, who lost his California license as a
result of his "nutritional" activities, does not wish to have further
legal difficulties.

Nittler also appears to be associated with the Natra-Bio Company of Marina Del Rey, California. This company distributes
"homeopathic alternatives to drugstore remedies," including 24
Natra-Bio Homeopathic Home Remedies each labeled with the
name of a symptom or disease. No. 503 is NERVOUSNESS; No.
516 is PROSTATE; No. 518 is BEDWETTING; and so on. Their use
is explained in a booklet written by Dr. Nittler and distributed by
the company for sale through health food stores.

• The Nutrition and Biomagnetic Seminar promises "a complete background in basic nutrition, all that is needed by a doctor
with no experience in Clinical Nutrition," in just one weekend.
The seminar is run by Richard Broeringmeyer, D.C., N.D., an
"associate" of Drs. Nittler and Evers, who lives in Murray, Ken-
tucky. According to Dr. Broeringmeyer, "magnetic energies" can
tell the doctor which organ is involved in the patient's problems

and what nutrients he needs. The seminar, which costs $125 or less, has been sponsored by the American Biomagnetic Association and Biomagnetic Internationale. Flyers for the seminar state that Dr. Broeringmeyer belongs to the International Academy of Preventive Medicine, the American Chiropractic Association Council on Nutrition, the Maryland State Homeopathic Medical Society, and the International College of Physicians and Surgeons (Homeopathic). He is also head of the International Biomagnetic Association and President of Health Industries, Inc. (which has the same address as Seroyal Brands of Mid America, a food supplement company). His wife and one son are also "chiropractic nutritionists."

The first issue of *Bioenergetics Magazine* (Richard Broeringmeyer, Ph.D., editor), published by the International Academy of Biomagnetic Medicine (same address as Health Industries), was distributed free-of-charge to all chiropractors in September 1980. Its contents include an ad for *Ultra Complete,* a "mega-vitamin—protein chelated mineral supplement" sold by Bioenergetics (same address), and an article by Dr. Broeringmeyer which concludes:

> If each of us would have perfect nutrition to produce the proper amount of energy with proper elimination there would be little if any disease and we could produce a super race. THERE IS REALLY NO DISEASE ONLY DEFICIENCIES CAUSING LOSS OF ELECTRO ENERGIES PRODUCING DISEASE AND EVENTUAL DEATH.

The number of chiropractors involved in nutrition schemes is not known to us, but is probably several thousand. Each of the above organizations, except for Dr. Nittler's, spends enough money each year advertising in journals and/or by direct mail to suggest that they have acquired sizable followings.

Naturopathy and Iridology

Naturopathy is a system of healing said to rely solely on "natural therapies." Naturopaths claim that the basic cause of disease is the violation of nature's laws. Diseases are viewed as the body's effort to purify itself, and cures result from "increasing the patient's vital force by ridding the body of toxins." Naturopathic treatment modalities include "natural food" diets, vitamins, herbs, tissue minerals, cell salts, manipulation, massage, remedial exercise, diathermy, colonic enemas, acupuncture, reflexology, hypnotherapy and homeopathy. Radiation may be used for diagnosis but not for treatment. Drugs are forbidden except for compounds that are components of body tissues.

Naturopaths, like chiropractors, believe that virtually all diseases are within the scope of their practice. They are licensed in seven states and the District of Columbia. The number of practitioners is unknown, but has been estimated to be a few thousand, most of whom practice in nonlicensing states. There may also be a few thousand chiropractors who practice naturopathy.

Prior to 1961, the doctor of naturopathy (N.D.) degree could be obtained at a number of chiropractic schools. Now it is available only from four schools of naturopathy. Training at these schools follows a pattern similar to that of chiropractic schools: two years of basic science courses and two years of clinical naturopathy. The schools are not accredited by any agency recognized by the United States Office of Education.

Iridology (also called iridiagnosis) is a system of diagnosis devised more than 100 years ago by Ignatz von Peczely, a Hungarian physician. It is based on the belief that each area of the body is represented by a corresponding area in the iris of the eye (the colored area surrounding the pupil). States of health and disease, as well as indications of past treatment, can supposedly be diagnosed from the color, texture and location of various pigment flecks in the eye.

A scientific test of iridology has been reported in the September 29, 1979 *Journal of the American Medical Association.* Three iridologists, including Bernard Jensen, D.C., the leading American proponent, examined photographs of the eyes of 143 persons in an attempt to determine which ones had kidney impairments. (Forty-eight had been medically diagnosed on the basis of creatinine clearance tests, and the rest had normal kidney function.) The three iridologists scored no better than chance.

Holistic Philosophy

Promoters of "holistic medicine" (also called "wholistic medicine") believe that illnesses should not be studied apart from the people who have them. Professional attention should therefore not be limited to current physical problems, but should also be directed toward emotional factors and lifestyles. Good physicians have always done this, but the holistic movement is now being promoted as *something new* by unscientific cultists, crusading laymen and a few hundred physicians. The promotion rests on an elaborate but loosely defined philosophy which has some basis in fact, but a close look will show that much of it is irrational.

Five themes appear central to the current philosophy of holistic medicine:

1. Individuals have primary responsibility for their health.
2. General measures, such as "reducing stress" and "correcting imbalances," can make people less susceptible to disease.
3. Medicine is too rigid and impersonal.
4. Medicine is just one healing art among many.
5. "Alternative" approaches, though indefinable, unendorsable and unproven, should be promoted vigorously.

Let's look at these themes more closely.

Something Extra?

It is well known to health scientists that smoking promotes cancer, that overeating and excessive alcohol intake are dangerous, that appropriate exercise is good for people, that use of safety belts can reduce the incidence of serious automobile injuries, etc. To the extent that holistic promoters persuade their followers to adopt better health practices, they can accomplish some good. But holistic promoters offer no useful addition to what good physicians have been doing all along.

Many holistic practitioners see disease as primarily caused by stresses and "imbalances." Although stress is a factor in many ailments, it is by no means clear that stress-reduction techniques advocated in the name of holism are actually effective in preventing disease. The concept of "imbalances" is even more fanciful. Acupuncturists claim to balance "life forces," chiropractors claim to balance spines, dubious dentists claim to balance "body chemistry," kinesiologists claim to balance muscles, and various other "healers" claim to balance people's spiritual, mental and physical "systems" to bring them "into harmony with nature." A common goal is a state of "wellness" that goes far beyond the absence of disease.

Holistic promoters tend to view nature as harmonious and benign. They depict primitive man as living in a utopian state which can be ours if we return to "natural" living. They are correct that many people feel negatively toward our health care system, but this is a very curious phenomenon. Polls show that most people are satisfied with their own medical care. Their antagonism is toward the "system"—which they view as overpriced or too self-serving. It is also true that more people are turning toward "alternative" methods. But disillusionment with scientific medicine is by no means the main reason for this (any more than dissatisfaction with astronomy is the primary cause of astrology's popularity). Many people have hopes and magical wishes that cannot possibly be satisfied by science.

Holistic proponents make a serious error by pretending that all of medicine is one system and then listing various others as separate but equal systems. They may call modern medicine "Western medicine" to distinguish it from "Eastern medicine." Or they may call it "allopathic medicine," a term coined almost two centuries ago by Samuel Hahnemann, the founder of homeopathy. In Hahnemann's day, allopathy included cupping, bloodletting and many other primitive methods then considered orthodox. Today, allopathy is no longer a school of thought. It includes all methods of treatment which are sensible, reliable and reproducible from one practitioner to another. Holistic advocates atttempt to reduce its significance by defining it as one approach. A wide variety of other approaches are then promoted as "alternatives."

Acupuncture defines the body according to systems with functions that have no relation to what is actually known about body physiology. The systems are said to be affected by color, weather, emotion and other factors. "Meridians" and acupuncture points on the surface of the body, which supposedly refer to internal organ functions, cannot actually be seen or measured. They are part of the mystical ancient Chinese way of looking at the body, health, disease and nature. It is claimed that stimulation of acupuncture points can benefit organ systems and return their functions to normal. The same claims are also made for *acupressure* (Shiatsu), but no needles are used. Acupuncture works by suggestion, somewhat like hypnosis, and can also produce enough pain to trigger release of the body's own morphine-like drugs (endorphins). Either of these mechanisms may produce temporary pain relief, but there is no evidence that acupuncture can affect the course of any physical illness. Many acupuncture patients have contracted hepatitis from contaminated needles.

When Dr. Herbert was in mainland China as a visiting professor, he was shown 10 operations performed under "acupuncture anesthesia." In every instance, the anethesiologist's chart showed that the patient had received significant pain-dulling medication before the operation.

Herbalism involves the use of thousands of substances whose chemical actions may not be known to the herbalists who use them. Herbs are promoted with the mystique of being "natural" and of possibly containing useful substances as yet undiscovered by science. Such promotion overlooks the fact that drug companies routinely test large numbers of naturally occurring substances and are quick to investigate new rumors about folk remedies. Many herbal remedies exert no pharmacological effect upon the body. Others contain potent drugs, some of which can be toxic or even lethal.

Homeopathy is a system of treatment which uses a wide variety of herbs, drugs and other chemicals in extremely tiny doses. It is based on the idea that if a substance can produce symptoms like those of an illness in healthy persons, a tiny amount of the substance can cure an illness in a sick person. When substances are so diluted that they could not possibly be effective against anything, homeopathic practitioners may still claim that an "essence" of the active ingredient exists even though the substance itself is no longer present. Homeopathy enjoyed some success during the 19th century when its methods (the equivalent of doing nothing) were less dangerous than some of the other treatments of that period. Today its use is utter nonsense.

Applied *kinesiology* is a system of diagnosis and treatment based on the notion that every organ dysfunction is accompanied by a specific weak muscle. Kinesiologists also claim that nutritional deficiencies, allergies and other adverse reactions to food substances can be detected by placing substances in the mouth so that the patient salivates. "Good" substances will lead to increased strength in specific muscles, whereas "bad" substances will cause specific weaknesses. Treatment of muscles diagnosed as "weak" may include special diets, food supplements, acupressure and/or spinal manipulation. Kinesiology was developed primarily by chiropractors but is being promoted to other practitioners as well.

Reflexology is a system of treatment which claims that pressure on the hand or foot can relieve the symptoms and remove the underlying cause of disease in other parts of the body. According to a prominent practitioner, reflexology has relieved liver trouble, anemia, deafness, falling hair, emphysema, cataracts, prostate trouble, heart disease, kidney trouble and a wide variety of other diseases and conditions. If you believe this, you will believe anything.

Polarity therapy supposedly "coordinates diet, exercise and techniques of body manipulation to increase and balance the flow of vital energy for the physical, emotional and mental well-being of the individual." According to Pierre Pannetier, director of the Polarity Center in Orange, California, "Love and understanding are the chief qualifications for applying the art . . . Teachers are the mere channels; everyone has the power to heal himself."

A common goal of holistic promoters is to find "the amounts of nutrients that will provide the utmost in health." Many use hair analysis and other questionable diagnostic tests. Most recommend high dosages of vitamins and minerals for the prevention and treatment of disease. There is no doubt that diet plays a role in the production of some diseases. Overweight is certainly a widespread problem, and some aspects of diet may someday prove to be related to the development of arteriosclerosis. But holistic promoters go far beyond what is scientifically valid.

Holistic Organizations

Practitioners who consider themselves "holistic" have been grouping into clinics that offer services and professional organizations which may enhance their status.

The International Academy of Preventive Medicine (IAPM) was founded in 1971 "to create an atmosphere conducive to open discussion of preventive medical measures among physicians, dentists, Ph.D.s and health-related professionals." It has about 850 members, almost all of whom are American. About 30 percent of them are dentists, 25 percent are medical doctors, 17 percent are osteopaths, and 12 percent are chiropractors. IAPM holds two national conferences each year and publishes a journal and a newsletter. According to its membership directory, "The Academy does not endorse any specific treatment or therapy, but in general, members . . . are vitally interested in two vital areas—prevention of chronic degenerative diseases and the relationship of medical nutrition to the prevention of disease and the maintenance of health." (Translation: It is a forum for questionable methods which operates by rules different from those of the scientific community.)

The International College of Applied Nutrition, a similar organization, has about 500 members.

The American Academy of Medical Preventics is "an educational society for health care professionals interested in the prevention and/or treatment of chronic degenerative diseases." One of its goals is "to insure the public awareness of alternative holistic methods of prevention and treatment." It has about 200 members, almost all of them medical doctors or osteopaths, whose "alternative" methods include chelation therapy, acupuncture and the use of megavitamins.

The American Holistic Medical Association (AHMA), formed in 1978, has a few hundred members, all of them medical or osteopathic physicians. Its major goals are "to establish standards for new concepts of therapy," to "evaluate and expand scientific medicine," and to educate professionals in the principles of "medicine of the whole person." It publishes a journal and a monthly newsletter, and sponsors week-long educational conferences three times a year. Subjects at the conferences have included: acupuncture, homeopathy, spiritual well-being, stress reduction, faith healing, rolfing (a method of "aligning" the body by vigorous manipulations), psychosynthesis, nontraditional methods of diagnosis, metaphysics, alignment through music, psycho-electronics, renewal and personal awakening, scientific medicine, and holistic treatment of inoperable cancer (by Dr. Contreras!). Most of the exhibitors at the meetings are promoters of questionable products and services.

Two things are remarkable about AHMA's meetings. First, a few of the invited speakers are reputable educators, including medical school deans, who are paid substantial sums to speak. Second, the meetings are endorsed for educational purposes by several major professional organizations.

To qualify for the "AMA Physician's Recognition Award," a physician must complete 150 hours of continuing education every three years. Sixty hours must be programs certified as "Category I" by an organization accredited by the Accreditation Council for Continuing Medical Education (ACCME). The purpose of the accreditation system is to ensure quality educational programs upon which physicians can rely. For the most part, the system is working well. Most accredited programs are sponsored by medical schools and teaching hospitals.

However, despite the questionable nature of most of its topics, AHMA is now accredited by ACCME and can give Category I credits for its programs. The meetings, and similar ones sponsored by other holistic organizations, have also received approval from dental, nursing and other professional organizations.

The Lehigh Valley Committee Against Health Fraud has suggested that lists be developed of treatment approaches and individuals whose lectures could not be certified for continuing education credit. But sponsoring organizations fear that creation of such lists would trigger expensive lawsuits. Some sponsors also maintain that since scientifically trained health professionals should be able to separate useful material from quackery, they do not need protection from questionable sources. Even if this were true (which it is not), the issue is not so simple. Do you think it serves any legitimate purpose to allow 40 hours of nonsense to be certified as 40 hours of health education? We strongly hope that ACCME develops the courage to stop accrediting groups which promote the questionable methods described in this book. If it does not, accreditation for continuing medical education will become meaningless.

During the summer of 1980, a meeting called "Cancer Dialogue '80" was widely advertised to health professionals by direct mail and by ads in reputable professional publications. Co-sponsored by AHMA and two other organizations, it was billed as "an innovative symposium" that would bring together many of the world's most prominent cancer specialists. The meeting was actually organized by the Omega Foundation, a school run by a Moslem sect and based in Lebanon Springs, New York, which specializes in mystical, cultural and "holistic" courses of study.

According to an article in *Medical World News*, eight prominent cancer experts agreed to participate in the program—for $2,000 apiece plus expenses—with the understanding that the other respected scientists known to them had agreed to come. They were not told that promoters of unscientific treatments would also make presentations at the meeting. Although these experts withdrew as soon as they learned the full structure of the meeting, people who answered the ads were not told of the program changes until a few days before the meeting took place. The meeting was also advertised to the public.

Three nurses from an Eastern Pennsylvania hospital, whose tumor department wasted its entire annual educational budget sending them to the meeting, reported that the program was dominated by advocates of questionable methods. The audience, which filled a large ballroom, contained many cancer patients—some in wheelchairs and on crutches—who obviously were looking for miracles. A list of laetrile and "metabolic" doctors was distributed at a table next to the one where certificates for continuing education credits were given out!

At the AHMA annual meeting in May 1981, the best-located booth was that of American Biologics, a major promoter of questionable remedies from laetrile to DMSO. Its president, Robert Bradford, is a convicted laetrile smuggler. Yet the seminar he gave on treating cancer with laetrile was certified for Category I credit. In addition to its "educational" goal, the American Holistic Medical Association may be aiming to protect its members from legal difficulty when they use questionable methods. According to a letter from an attorney published in the AHMA newsletter:

> There is case authority that suggests that if a physician can show that he has used a method of treatment which is approved by at least a respectable minority of medical opinion, the burden of sustaining an action against the physician

shifts to the accuser . . . to demonstrate that the method in question was applied in a negligent manner. In the event that the AHMA were to establish a sound membership base and establish official position on various types of treatment modalities, this provision might come into play and be used to the benefit of physicians who were employing alternative therapy sanctioned by the Association.

At one time in the past, the holistic label had a valuable and specific meaning. Today, however, it has become a banner around which all manner of questionable practitioners are rallying. It appears to us that the concept of holism has been irretrievably corrupted by confused practitioners and promoters of quackery. *The word "holistic" and its associated slogans should be abandoned by scientific practitioners.*

If professionals who believe in science could organize half as effectively as the "unscientific community" described in this book, nutritional quackery would be much more difficult to sell and the health consumer would be much better protected.

Chapter 7

The "Natural-Organic" Ripoff

Foods labeled "organic," "organically grown" or "natural" usually cost more than "regular" or "conventionally grown" foods. Sometimes they cost twice as much—or more. Are they worth their extra cost? Are they any different from foods not so labeled?

Let us begin our inquiry by asking what the "organic" labels mean. In December 1972, New York State Attorney General Louis Lefkowitz held a public hearing on this matter. Robert Rodale, one of the nation's most active "organic" promoters, testified as follows:

Organically grown food is food grown without pesticides; grown without artificial fertilizers; grown in soil whose humus content is increased by the additions of organic matter; grown in soil whose mineral content is increased by the applications of natural mineral fertilizers; has not been treated with preservatives, hormones, antibiotics, etc.

Let's look closely at the components of this definition to see if they make sense.

"Without Pesticides"

This part of the definition relates to the fear many people have that pesticides threaten their health. Organic promoters *imply* two things: (1) that the use of pesticides is bad and dangerous; and (2) that foods grown under "organic" conditions will contain no pesticides. Although the Rodale definition does not actually state that organically grown foods are *free* of pesticides, it is clear that many retailers make this claim. Vincent White, Confidential Investigator for the New York State Bureau of Consumer Frauds and Protection, spoke on this point at the Lefkowitz hearing. After visiting 25 stores as a prospective buyer of organic foods, he reported that "the general consensus was that they were pesticide free."

But they are not. Over the years, *many laboratories have found little difference in the level of pesticide residues between foods which are labeled "organic" and those which are not.*

73

For example, the New York State Department of Agriculture and Markets, which has been comparing "organic" and regular foods since 1972, has found "no significant differences" in the incidence or level of pesticides. In 1978, researchers from Wayne State and Michigan State University tested 10 brands of bread, 5 from health food stores and 5 from supermarkets. All 10 contained traces of pesticides. In 1979, Agriscience Laboratories, a Los Angeles firm which does pesticide testing for government agencies as well as for private companies, analyzed 28 samples of "organic" fruits and vegetables from health food stores and 14 nonorganic samples from supermarkets. No overall difference in pesticide levels was found between the two groups of foods. Only 2 of the 42 samples were free of pesticides. One of these was from a supermarket.

Thus, if you buy "organic" labeled foods in the hope of avoiding pesticides, you are unlikely to be successful. But don't let this trouble you. Government agencies keep watch on our food supplies to be sure they are safe to eat. The pesticide content of today's food is not a threat to our health. The amounts of pesticides found in our foods are extremely small. They would not even be detectable if it were not for the exquisite sensitivity of modern measuring equipment which can measure some substances in parts per trillion! Moreover, pesticides have a greater margin of safety than many other substances found naturally in foods which we eat all the time without worrying about them.

"Without Artificial Fertilizers"

Organic promoters suggest that "natural" fertilizers are better able to nourish plants and that they result in more nutritious foods. They also suggest that natural fertilizers contain, or might contain, some ingredient found in nature but lacking in artificial fertilizers. These ideas are good sales gimmicks, but nothing more. From the plant's point of view, it makes no difference where its food comes from. Chemicals are taken up and used by the plant in their inorganic chemical state no matter whether they are fed to the plant in manure, compost or manufactured fertilizer. All the plant cares about is whether it has enough food. If it does, it will grow. If it does not, it will not grow.

Experiments conducted at the Michigan Experimental Station for 10 years, at the U.S. Plant, Soil and Nutrition Laboratory at Cornell University for 25 years, and at the British Experimental Farm for 34 years, all indicate that there are no differences in major nutrient content whether foods are grown on soils fed with animal or synthetic plant foods. The amount of vitamin C in apples, for example, cannot be made equal to that in oranges by the addition of any amount of fertilizer. This is because nutritional content (other than minerals) is controlled by genes (the plant's heredity).

Fertilizers may influence the mineral composition of plants. The iodine content, for example, may vary with the iodine content of the soil, and the same may be true of other elements such as zinc, cobalt and selenium. But these variations are rarely significant in the diet.

The fact that mineral content of soil can affect mineral content of plants encourages the organic food industry to suggest that its recommended fertilizers are the best way to supply minerals. "After all," they say, "we return to nature what belongs to nature. Animals that eat plants nourished by soil return the elements to the soil via their manure. Nothing is lost." This, however, is faulty reasoning. If a soil is deficient in a nutrient, use of manure from animals fed from that soil is the surest way to guarantee that the nutrient will remain missing. The best way to insure proper plant growth is to determine by analysis what the soil needs and to add the needed chemicals.

At the New York State hearing, Dr. Mark Schwartz, Rodale Press's nutritionist, was asked whether Rodale publications generally take the position that organic foods are nutritionally superior to regular foods. He replied, "I don't think that organic foods are any different from the foods that we ordinarily eat. The thing we are talking about is the method of producing these foods." In other words, "organically grown" foods are neither different nor better!

Even if its leaders publicly deny making claims of nutritional superiority, however, there is no question that the industry as a whole suggests to its customers that its methods nourish plants better and therefore will nourish people better. To quote further from Investigator White's testimony:

Q. Did you find a pattern of representation existed among the stores which you visited as to the virtues of organic food?

A. Yes, sir, the general consensus was that they were . . . more nutritious and that they would be healthier in the long run if consumed by an individual.

Q. Were any examples given to you of what would happen if you purchased organic food in regard to illness? Was that stressed?

A. Yes, there were a few establishments who told me that if you are a little heavy, and you eat organically grown food, you might lose some weight or might be free of diabetes.

"Additions of Organic Matter"

The implication here is that organic matter *alone* conditions soil best for plants. It has long been standard agricultural practice to plow crop residues and "green manuring crops" back into the soil. This makes the soil easier to work and can improve the seed-bed for the coming crop. This practice works well in combination with the use of fertilizers. Composts and animal manures may also help the physical characteristics of the soil. In fact, there are times when the so-called "mulching" process is needed and highly advantageous. Scientific farmers can easily determine and use whatever their soil needs. Incidentally, research scientists can grow vigorous, healthy plants "hydroponically"— with no soil at all, just chemical nutrients added to water. This method is not yet practical for large-scale farming, but it highlights the lack of logic in the above organic myth.

Low availability and high distribution costs make it clear that the world cannot rely on animal-produced fertilizers to grow its food. It takes 20 pounds of manure to supply the same amount of nutrients as one pound of synthetic fertilizer. More often than not, the wastes from cows, horses and chickens accumulate at great distances from food-growing areas. It is expensive to collect and haul manures great distances and then spread them on fields.

Manure has another disadvantage. It can contaminate plants with Salmonella germs which can cause serious diarrheal illness (dysentery). Manure can also spread intestinal parasites.

"Not Treated with Preservatives, Hormones, Antibiotics"

Here the organic and natural food promoters suggest that *all* food additives are bad. But they don't tell you that without the use of additives, it would be impossible to feed large populations. They also don't mention that preservatives have been used for centuries to prevent foods from spoiling. The salting of meat and the pickling of cucumbers are familiar examples. Hormones are present naturally in *all* animals and plants. Antibiotics are not used to treat foods, but are valuable in controlling diseases of farm animals—some of which are dangerous to humans. Some antibiotics which are fed to farm animals travel through their intestines without getting into their meat. Those that do get into meat are destroyed by cooking.

Today there are some 2,800 substances intentionally added to foods. It is the responsibility of the FDA to judge the safety of these substances, and a great deal of attention has been paid to this matter. Food additives, particularly those introduced in the past 15 years, have survived rigid testing procedures not applied to the great majority of natural products. These tests must prove that the additive is not only safe, but performs an important function.

Additives make up less than one percent of our food. The most widely used are sugar, salt and corn syrup—all found naturally. These three, plus citric acid (found naturally in oranges and lemons), baking soda, vegetable colors, mustard and pepper, account for 98 percent by weight of all food additives used in this country.

Most additives are used—in tiny quantities—to enhance food colors and flavors. Most people want their food to look appealing. A ripe orange that loses its characteristic color as a result of temperature variation may be perfectly edible and nutritious. But people who don't think it "looks right" won't eat it. Food dyes are used to correct this situation. Taste is equally important. Variety keeps our diet interesting, but there is simply not enough natural flavoring around to satisfy our demanding taste buds. For example, there is not enough natural vanilla in the whole world to flavor the ice cream we eat in this country in a year. So we make synthetic vanillin, the flavoring substance found in vanilla extract.

Additives also perform vital functions in food preservation and enrichment. The World Health Organization estimates that almost a quarter of the food produced is lost each year before it gets into consumer hands as a result of infestation by insects and rodents and because of spoilage. Food additives slow down deterioration considerably, and as a result, make the food supply more plentiful. Antibiotic preservatives prevent spoilage by bacteria, molds, fungi and yeast. They also extend shelf-life and protect natural food color or flavor. Antioxidants delay or prevent rancidity or enzymatic browning.

Calcium propionate, which is used to prevent bread from getting moldy, offers an especially penetrating illustration of the health food industry's lack of logic about additives. This chemical is normally produced, as well as used, in the human body. Leaving it out of bread will do the consumer no good whatsoever. It will, however, result in a lot of moldy bread being thrown out in the garbage. And, as we point out in Chapter 2, people who eat a Swiss cheese sandwich consume enough calcium propionate from one ounce of natural cheese to preserve two loaves of bread.

These facts should make it clear that sweeping general attacks on food additives make no sense at all. The only proper way to evaluate food additives is to do so individually. Scientists do this, of course. FDA scientists, for example, set careful tolerance levels in foods and conduct frequent "market basket" studies wherein foods from 18 regions of the United States are purchased and analyzed.

"Etc."

The term "etc." is not defined. Presumably, this allows the definition to be expanded at will to keep pace with the imagination of "organic" producers. As Investigator White indicated at the Lefkowitz hearing, the "organic" label is not confined to fruits and vegetables:

Q. Did any specific food example stick in your mind, Mr. White?

A. Yes, the eggs. I asked in several establishments why it is necessary to charge the inflated price for the eggs and I was told that these eggs were produced by organically grown chickens, that these chickens were free of hormones and they were allowed to roam free with the rooster . . .

Q. Did you come upon a store that was selling fish?

A. Yes . . .

Q. Did the man selling fish tell you why it was organic?

A. Yes, he claimed that it was caught in the pollution-free, mineral-rich Atlantic Ocean.

A team of scientists appointed by the U.S. Department of Agriculture (USDA) to study "organic farming" concluded recently that there is no universally accepted definition of the term. The study team report, issued in 1980, states:

. . . the organic movement represents a spectrum of practices, attitudes and philosophies. On the one hand are those organic practitioners who would not use chemical fertilizers or pesticides under any circumstances. These producers hold rigidly to their purist philosophy. At the other end of the spectrum, organic farmers espouse a more flexible approach. While striving to avoid the use of chemical fertilizers and pesticides, these practitioners do not rule them out entirely. Instead, when absolutely necessary, some fertilizers and also herbicides are very selectively and sparingly used as a second line of defense. Nevertheless, these farmers, too, consider themselves to be organic farmers. Failure to recognize that the organic farming movement is distributed over a spectrum can often lead to serious misconceptions.

It certainly can! Rodale's definition is not just meaningless and misleading. Many members of the "industry" consider themselves "organic" whether they actually follow the definition or merely do the best they can.

Undaunted by these realities, the USDA Study Team recommended that certification programs be established "to assure that organically produced foods are properly labeled" and that local USDA representatives should help organic producer associations develop criteria for certification standards!

Taste

Three factors affect the taste of fruits and vegetables: (1) their genetic make-up; (2) how ripe they are when harvested; and (3) how fresh they are when eaten. "Organic" food advocates claim that their products taste better. They claim that since their produce comes from small farms, it is more likely to be sold locally in fresh condition. They also claim that supermarket produce is bred for shipping and keeping qualities rather than for flavor.

These claims were scientifically tested by research at the University of Florida. In this experiment, 20 men and women, ages 18 to 60, met several times a week for 3 months to compare 25 "health" foods with their supermarket cousins. Color, flavor, texture, odor and general acceptance were rated. None of the "health" foods was found to be superior on the basis of general acceptance. However, many of the regular foods were rated as better for color, flavor, texture and general acceptance. Regular foods that were scored higher than health foods by the panel included dried apples, apple juice, applesauce, cashews, cereal, Swiss cheese, coconut, corn chips, ice cream, mayonnaise with tomato, peanut butter, sesame chips and tomato juice. The only health food qualities which were scored higher than those of regular foods were the odors of apple butter and pizza and the color of ketchup.

Cost

Many studies have shown that foods labeled "organic" cost more than conventionally grown foods. In 1972, for example, the U.S. Department of Agriculture compared prices in the District of Columbia. Here is what they found:

Comparison of Regular and "Organic" Food Prices

	SUPERMARKET		HEALTH Food Store	NATURAL Food Store
	"Regular" Department	"Organic" Department		
Canned apple juice, qt.	.29	.65	.75	.51
Dried peaches, lb.	.73	1.32	1.68	1.55
Corn meal, lb.	.14	.30	.44	.21
Honey, lb.	.55	.79	1.05	.50
Cucumbers, lb.	.19	.79	.69	.57
Total of above 5 items	1.90	3.85	4.61	3.34
"Market basket" of 29 standard foods	11.00	20.30	21.90	17.80

These prices, of course, are from the Good Old Days. However, the most interesting thing about the table is the price difference between regular and "organic" foods in the same supermarket. What do you think an on-the-ball store manager would do if he ran out of organic cucumbers and had plenty of the regular variety on hand (especially if he were aware that there is no basic difference between the two products anyway)?

The Appeal for "Consumer Protection"

Without doubt, the typical 50-100 percent markup has led many enterprising merchants to label regular foods "organic." Calling this practice deceptive, promoters of "real" organic food have been asking government agencies to "protect" their customers from "fake" organic food. Ignoring the fact that "real" organic food is identical or inferior to regular food, they suggest that their customers should be able to get "what they think they are paying for"—that is, foods produced by "genuine" organic methods.

Rodale Press has designed a "certification" program whereby farmers who follow its suggested methods are given labels which indicate that their methods meet Rodale standards. Once the labels are given to the farmers, however, there is no practical way to supervise how the labels are used.

Organic certification proposals could be regarded as quite humorous except for the fact that some government officials have taken them seriously. Laws establishing organic "standards" have actually been passed in Oregon, New Hampshire and California. In Texas, the U.S. Office of Economic Opportunity has offered technical assistance so that "poor farmers can raise their incomes enough through organic farming to stay on the land." Because organic farming requires more labor to achieve essentially the *same products as regular farming,* however, such "assistance" may actually cause the farmers to work harder for less produce and less profit.

Back to "Nature"

The word "natural" has become a magic sales gimmick. But its definitions by promoters are even more meaningless than those of the word "organic." Even beer and tobacco are being boosted for their supposed natural qualities!

To further our inquiry, let's look at the definition of "natural foods" presented to the Federal Trade Commission by Annette Dickinson when she was lobbyist for the Council for Responsible Nutrition, a Washington-based group which represents manufacturers and distributors of food supplements sold through health food stores:

1. The source must be living plants and animals. Thus salt, naturally occurring sodium chloride, may be considered natural.
2. The concept applies only to post-harvest treatment of food.
3. Natural fruits and vegetables are harvested ripe, so that the indigenous flavor, color and nutritional value are fully developed, except that climacteric fruits, such as bananas, may be harvested before ripening.
4. The inedible portions of natural foods may be removed. This includes peeling or seeding of some fruits and vegetables, shelling of nuts, removal of chaff and hull from grains, etc.
5. The edible portions may be processed only by certain physical or mechanical methods or by fermentation. Specific processes are limited to the following:

   A. The product may be cut into smaller portions.
   B. Fruits and vegetables may be pressed to express their juices.
   C. Oils may be expressed from seeds and other source materials by pressing.
   D. Grains may be rolled, cut or ground. Whole grain flours and meals are natural. When whole grains are separated into their component parts, the components will not be considered natural unless they have a nutrient density at least as great as that of whole grain.

In the case of whole wheat, the effect will be that whole wheat flour, bran and germ will qualify as natural, while white flour will not.

E. Eggs are natural products, as are yolks and whites used separately.

F. The refining of sugar beets, sugar cane, etc., to produce highly purified sugars is inappropriate for natural foods and the resulting sugars are not natural. This applies to molasses and to brown or "raw" sugars as well as white sugars or syrups. The only sugars occurring in nature in a form approximating their commercial form are honey and maple syrup.

G. Whole milk is a natural product. When separated into skim milk and cream, the resulting products are also natural. Dairy products may be pasteurized only to the extent required by public health laws. They may not be subjected to more severe heat to extend shelf life. They may be homogenized, churned or fermented.

H. Natural foods which are fluid or have a high moisture content may be concentrated but not subject to extreme dehydration, as in dry milk, instant coffee and freeze-dried vegetables.

I. Traditional methods of sun-drying are appropriate for natural foods such as spices, fruits and teas, provided no additives are used.

J. Refrigeration and freezing are appropriate . . .

K. Natural foods may be heated to the extent necessary for preservation and/or palatability. Dry heat such as roasting of nuts and baking of bread are acceptable. Moist heat treatment such as blanching, boiling or steaming are appropriate. Frying is not, since this adds oil or fat to a food.

L. Traditional methods of smoking, drying and curing meats are appropriate if they do not involve the use of additives.

M. Fermentation is appropriate, whether accomplished by naturally occurring organisms or by added cultures.

N. Micro-organisms approved by the FDA for use in food are themselves a natural food.

6. Natural food may consist of a single ingredient or a combination of ingredients provided each is a natural food.

7. No artificial or synthetic ingredient may be used.

8. The color, flavor and nutritional value should be indigenous to the food or its basic ingredients. Added purified flavors, colors and nutrients are not appropriate . . .

Thomas H. Jukes, Ph.D., a prominent nutritionist and agricultural expert who is Professor of Medical Physics at the University of California in Berkeley, has carefully analyzed the above definition and finds it "irrational and full of inconsistencies." In point 1, after declaring that natural foods must come from live plants and animals, Ms. Dickinson stretches to include table salt, which comes from neither. Point 3 includes ripe fruits in the category of natural, but excludes most unripe ones. Presumably some magical change occurs during ripening to convert unnatural fruits and vegetables into natural ones.

Point 5 goes the other way. Sugar is refined by a process of crystallization which removes dirt and other inedible substances. The end result is pure sucrose—unchanged by crystallization—the very same sucrose that is found in fruits and vegetables. Pure sucrose contains no additives, pesticide residues or other "artificial" or synthetic ingredients. But according to Ms. Dickinson, the purification process makes it unnatural. Natural honey, as defined by her, may contain allergy-causing substances and disease-causing bacteria. But pasteurization, which inactivates both, makes the end product unnatural.

According to 5G and 5H, removing cream from milk leaves a natural product (skim milk), but removing water from milk creates an unnatural one (powdered milk). The separation of cream also removes vitamin A, but point 8 states that replacing the lost vitamin A by fortification makes the milk unnatural.

Item 5L states that traditional methods of smoking meat are natural if they do not involve the use of additives. However, the residue of the smoke itself is an additive that may even cause cancer. Point 5K ignores the fact that processing by heat is necessary for certain foods, such as soybeans, to inactivate enzyme inhibitors and thus make them digestible. Point 8 excludes the addition of vitamins and minerals to foods, ignoring, for example, the public health value of iodized salt in preventing goiter. Item 5J allows freezing, but 5H forbids freeze-drying. And so on.

The FTC Reacts

Ms. Dickinson's definition of "natural" was presented to the FTC during a rulemaking proceeding that began in November 1974 in response to the turmoil surrounding advertising claims for many types of food products. Claims for "organic," "natural" and "health" foods were among them. The FTC noted originally that the three terms were not clearly defined and were also used interchangeably by both sellers and buyers of these products. The original FTC staff proposal included a ban on the terms, "organic," "natural," "organically grown" and "naturally grown."

Commissioner William D. Dixon presided over the FTC inquiry. In January 1978, after several periods of public comment, including 50 days of live testimony by interested parties, Mr. Dixon issued his findings. Foods labeled "organic" or "natural" are not safer or more nutritious than their ordinary counterparts. Indeed, in many instances, "natural" foods may be *less* safe or nutritious than foods which have been fortified or highly processed.

Although Mr. Dixon reached the correct *scientific* conclusions, his *political* conclusion was that public confusion "points more toward the need for definition to govern use of the terms than a total ban on their use." The term "health food" should be banned as inherently misleading, he thought, but the terms "organic" and "natural" should be officially defined by the FTC. Despite its inconsistencies, Ms. Dickinson's submission was regarded by Mr. Dixon as "among the most constructive received" and could well "form the basis for a final solution."*

Later in 1978, the FTC staff issued its recommendations for a final rule. No food could be advertised as a "health food," but the term "health food store" would still be permitted. "Organic" and "natural" would be redefined by the FTC. The organic definition would be similar to that of Rodale Press, and "natural" would mean "minimal processing." But in 1980, the full Commission

---

*Recently Ms. Dickinson sent the following letter to Dr. Barrett: "... There are indeed some defects in the definition of 'natural foods' I submitted to the FTC several years ago, but I don't agree [with Dr. Jukes] in every case about where the defects lie. It was never intended as a final definition, but was simply one step in the long process of seeking consensus on a feasible approach ... I had hoped that FTC would convene a panel of experts to cover the specifics of a definition, but that was never done. My definition was developed rather at the last minute, simply to serve as a skeleton which could be dismantled or built upon by the staff. The process was bogging down for lack of a tangible target for discussion, so I offered a useful target. As it turned out, the Presiding Officer found it useful, and the staff re-worked it considerably following publication of the Presiding Officer's report. In any case, my specific definition was submitted on my own behalf, as an individual, and not on behalf of the Council. I had testified at the hearings on behalf of the Council, but they (perhaps wisely) were not comfortable with pursuing the matter beyond that point ..."

decided not to prohibit health food claims or adopt standards for organic foods. It also instructed the staff to consider further the standards for "natural" foods.

In our opinion, government definition of any of the health food industry's slogans will be interpreted by the public as an endorsement of the mythology that surrounds the slogans. Shoppers are not going to be reminded of the FTC's *scientific* conclusions. They will merely see the labels and be invited to pay higher prices for "superior" products.

There is also the question of enforceability. No definitions of the words "natural" and "organic" can be devised that are logical or consistent with scientific facts. "Minimum processing" is indefinable, and "organically grown" foods cannot be distinguished from their conventional counterparts. Enforcement of intangible "standards" can lead only to endless arguments and a waste of government resources. As this book goes to press, it appears that the FTC may abandon its food advertising rule entirely.

Overview

Two hundred years ago, the average family in the Western world had to spend most of its time grubbing a meager living from the soil. The lack of fertilizer, the presence of pests that demolished crops, and the absence of knowledge about plant breeding, all combined to keep most people hungry. Then chemists discovered that plants were actually nourished by inorganic chemicals. Phosphate, potash, nitrate and ammonia were needed. They could come either from the breakdown of manure by soil bacteria, or from rock phosphate, inorganic potash, nitrates and ammonia salts. The agricultural revolution was on. Farmers became able to feed more and more city folk.

A century ago, farmers were helpless against the fungus blight which turned their potatoes into a black slime. As a result, one million people starved to death during the Irish potato famine. Pesticides to control the blight were not yet available.

As agricultural knowledge increased by leaps and bounds, farming became increasingly more scientific. Plant and animal breeding gave us fine new strains of grains, vegetables, fruits, poultry, pigs and cattle. More efficient fertilizers and a wide variety of pesticides were developed. Thanks to these advances, rare delicacies became commonplace.

The new chemical methods required careful regulation to see that farmers used them properly. Pure food laws were passed to make sure that only insignificant traces of unwanted pesticide residues were present in foods. These laws appear to be working well. There has not been one case of illness in America which can be attributed to a *scientific* agricultural procedure. In contrast, in countries where "organic" fertilizers (such as human waste) are used, food poisoning from disease organisms is quite common.

As scientific agriculture developed, so did methods of processing, preserving and distributing foods.

Against this 200-year background of fantastic scientific progress have emerged voices of quackery who cry that our food supply is neither safe nor nutritious. They either ignore or fail to understand scientific thought. They profit greatly by frightening the public into buying their ideas, their publications and their overpriced or unnecessary "health" products.

Many Americans, worried about pollution and flooded with misleading information in talk shows and publications, are responding to the quacks. Despite the fact that "organic" and "natural" foods can neither be defined meaningfully nor told apart from "regular" foods, many people are willing to pay more for them. Americans now spend more than a *billion* dollars a year for them. But the ultimate irony is that the organic-natural-health food industry, which itself preys on confusion and false hopes, may actually succeed in getting our government to set "standards" for its misleading slogans. Such legal endorsement would encourage the public to purchase "genuine" fakes—whose only extra is extra cost.

The organic-natural-health food lobby is clever and well organized. Let us hope that someday, government officials who are pressured by this lobby will see clearly who needs protection and from whom. Instead of protecting an industry which misleads consumers, our government should educate the public. And since the slogans of this industry cannot be accurately defined, their commercial use should be outlawed.

Chapter 8

Prominent Promoters

There have always been food fads. If you look hard enough, you could probably find historical expressions of concern about almost every item in the human diet. Foods are highly susceptible to rumor, and rumor promotes food faddism. Although the development of science has the potential to curb faddism, the parallel development of mass communication has enabled faddists to reach vast numbers of potential followers.

"Nature" Salesmen

Sylvester Graham (1794-1851) mixed religious fanaticism with a zeal for the natural, "uncomplicated" life. "The simpler, plainer and more natural the food," said Graham, "the more healthy, vigorous and long-lived will be the body." Among his prohibited foods were salt and other condiments (these and sexual excesses caused insanity), cooked vegetables (against God's law) and chicken pies (caused cholera). His most vigorous attacks were against "unnatural" substances such as meat, white flour products and water consumed at mealtime. Although Graham's health petered out at the age of 57, his spirit remains with us in the cracker that bears his name.

John Harvey Kellogg (1852-1943) supposedly ate his way through medical school on a diet of apples and graham crackers. He belonged to a Seventh-day Adventist group which had founded a religious colony and health sanitarium at Battle Creek, Michigan. It is said that he and his brother Will were the first men to make a million dollars from food faddism. Under Dr. Kellogg's leadership, the Battle Creek Sanitarium attracted large numbers of wealthy clients whose intestines he "detoxified" with enemas and high-fiber diets. In an effort to provide a dried product upon which his clients could exercise their teeth without breaking them, Kellogg hit upon the idea of a corn flake. By 1899, the flakes had evolved into a cereal-based company that had many competitors. One was Charles W. Post, a former Kellogg patient, who ground up wheat and barley loaves, called his product "grape nuts" and marketed it as a cure for appendicitis, malaria, consumption and loose teeth. Thus were the humble beginnings of today's two giant cereal manufacturers, the Kellogg Company and the Post Division of General Foods.

Horace Fletcher (1849-1919) was one of the few faddists to achieve some scientific recognition for this work. Grossly overweight and in poor health at the age of 40, he retired from business and sought "cures" throughout the world. After reading books "only to find that no two authors agreed," he finally "determined to consult Mother Nature herself for direction." Reasoning that "if Nature had given us personal responsibility it was not hidden away in the dark folds and coils of the [intestines] where we could not control it," he decided that the mouth held the key to the whole situation. Extremely thorough chewing—later termed "Fletcherizing"—was the key to good health. Using this method, he lost more than 60 pounds and (because of the weight loss) felt much better.

Although he didn't look it, Fletcher had always been an exceptionally strong individual. When he demonstrated his prowess at Yale University and elsewhere, people attributed his strength to his dietary habits. Fletcherizing, which was quite tedious, actually helped some people to eat less and therefore suffer less from the effects of overeating. (Today we call such maneuvers to eat less "behavior modification.") But as Fletcher's enthusiasm for his own theories increased, he gradually cut down further on the amount of food he ate and sometimes fasted for several days at a time. He died at Battle Creek Sanitarium, probably as a result of malnutrition.

Bernarr Macfadden (1868-1955) was the first faddist to use mass media techniques to amass a fortune. At age 18, well-muscled as a result of a 3-year exercise program, he launched his career as a teacher of "physical culture." Pupils were sparse, but he survived by selling bodybuilding gadgets and posing (almost nude) for pictures. *Physical Culture* magazine, which he began publishing in 1896, was a great success. The number of subscribers reached 100,000 within two years and eventually passed one million.

Two themes ran through almost every article in the magazine. One was that medical science should be rejected in favor of "natural" methods. The other was a special dietary program which included fasting. Within the next two decades, Macfadden published more than 20 books including a 5-volume *Encyclopedia of Physical Culture* containing "complete instruction for the cure of all diseases through physcultopathy." He also began other magazines—including *True Story, True Experiences,* and *True Detec-*

tive—all of which promoted eccentric health schemes and allowed advertisements for questionable methods of health care.

As medical science developed, Macfadden's influence gradually faded away. His place in the public spotlight was taken by others whose nonsense sounded more scientific.

One "Expert" After Another

Gayelord Hauser (1895-   ) promised to add years to your life with five wonder foods: skim milk, brewer's yeast, wheat germ, yogurt and blackstrap molasses. His book, *Look Younger, Live Longer,* led the bestseller list in 1951, the same year that 25 copies were seized by the FDA when they accompanied a shipment of blackstrap molasses. The court readily agreed that the molasses was misbranded by many false claims in the book. D. C. Jarvis, a physician, wrote that body alkalinity was the principal threat to American health and that honey and apple cider vinegar were the antidotes. False claims in his book were the basis for an FDA seizure of a product called "Honegar." Melvin Page, D.D.S., who warned that milk was an underlying cause of cancer, persuaded many of his followers to stop drinking it or giving it to their children. Thus came one faddist after another, each with his own brand of fear and magic.

Adolphus Hohensee (1901-1967) began his training in nutrition by taking a job as a soda jerk. After dabbling in real estate (with time in jail for mail fraud) and the field of transportation (during which time he was arrested for passing bad checks), he resumed his education. In 1943, he acquired an Honorary Degree of Doctor of Medicine from a non-accredited school and followed this with Doctor of Naturopathy degrees from two schools which he did not attend. In 1946, he acquired a chiropractic license in the state of Nevada.

A master showman, Hohensee could lecture for hours about the terrible American diet that he claimed would stagnate the blood, corrode the blood vessels, erode the kidneys and clog the intestines. Most people had intestinal worms, he said, that (fortunately) could be cured by his special cleansing diet. He promised a long life to those who consumed his wonder products. Repeated prosecution by the FDA made him more cautious about selling his products during lectures, but his promotion of the gamut of food myths sent his audiences flocking into nearby health food stores whose shelves just happened to be well-stocked with his product line. In 1955, alert reporters caught Hohensee eating a meal of forbidden foods after one of his lectures. Beginning in 1962, he served 18 months in prison for selling honey with false claims. But neither of these setbacks dampened his enthusiasm or that of his loyal followers.

Lelord Kordel (1904-   ), author of 19 books, recommends high-protein foods, lecithin ("the miracle nutrient") and high-dosage vitamin and mineral supplements for everyone. According to court records, he began producing and marketing supplements in 1941, operating under various trade names. In 1946, he was convicted of misbranding and fined $4,000. One product in the case was "Gotu Kola," an herbal tablet said to restore youth and "produce erect posture, sharp eyes, velvety skin, limbs of splendid proportions, deep chest, firm bodies, gracefully curved hips, flat abdomens" and even "pleasing laughter." Thirteen other products were falsely claimed to be effective against various conditions including heart disease, liver troubles, tuberculosis, bone infections and impotence.

Kordel had a brush with the FTC in 1957 and two more with the FDA in 1961. In 1963, when he was president of Detroit Vital Foods, Inc., products shipped by the company were found to be misbranded because they were accompanied by Kordel publications which falsely claimed that nutritional products could treat practically all diseases. After the appeals process was ended in 1971, Kordel was fined $10,000 and served one year in prison. Current catalogues from Vital Foods, Inc., describe him as "America's leading vitamin and diet expert" and claim that he "has never been ill."

The Consultant

Carlton Fredericks (1910-   ) is described on some of the covers of books he has written as "America's Foremost Nutritionist." According to the FDA, however, he has had virtually no nutrition or health science training. He graduated from the University of Alabama in 1931 (under his original name: Harold Frederick Caplan) with a major in English and a minor in political science. His only science courses were two hours of physiology and eight hours of elementary chemistry. He had various jobs until 1937 when he began to write advertising copy for the U.S. Vitamin Corporation and to give sales talks, adopting the title of "nutrition educator."

Records of the Magistrates' Court of New York City show that Fredericks began diagnosing patients and prescribing vitamins for their illnesses. After investigation by agents of the New York State Department of Education, Fredericks was charged with unlawful practice of medicine. In 1945, after pleading guilty, he paid a fine of $500 (rather than spend 3 months in jail) and joined the rolls of those with criminal convictions in connection with nutrition frauds.

Fredericks then enrolled in New York University's School of Education and received a master's degree in 1949 and a night school Ph.D. (in communications) in 1955 without having taken a single course in nutrition. The topic for his doctoral thesis was *A Study of the Responses of a Group of Adult Female Listeners to a Series of Educational Radio Programs.* These were his own radio programs—broadcast on New York City's WOR and distributed at times to other stations. The WOR broadcasts alone have been reported to generate more than 10,000 letters a week! As far as we know, Fredericks still has no educational qualifications that would make him an expert in the science of nutrition.

According to an article in *The Reporter* magazine, Fredericks was listed as "Chief Consultant" to Foods Plus, Inc., a vitamin company which ran into trouble with the FDA. In 1960, more than 200,000 bottles of the firm's food supplement preparations were seized as misbranded because literature accompanying them contained false claims that the preparations were useful in treating dozens of diseases.

The *Reporter* article also states that in 1961, an investigation by the Federal Communications Commission concluded that Fredericks had a contract with Foods Plus to turn over all mail received as a result of public appearances so that Foods Plus could use the names in the promotion and sale of its products. Fredericks terminated his relationship with Foods Plus in 1962, shortly after the FDA again charged the company with misbranding 42 products. The judge who decided this case in 1965 concluded that Fredericks had been telling a vast radio audience that vitamins and minerals can be used to treat more than 50 problems including arthritis, epilepsy, multiple sclerosis and even "lack of mental resistance to house-to-house salesmen." Fredericks' former contract with Foods Plus, the court ruled, made his questionable claims part of the company's product labeling. As an expert witness in the court case, Dr. Victor Herbert described Fredericks as a "charlatan." The defense attorney objected, but after Dr. Herbert read to the court the dictionary definition of charlatan, the objection was overruled.

Fredericks is one of the originators of the crusade to discredit sugar. He has deftly channeled this single theme into a number of variations which reflect and exploit current public concerns about alcoholism, emotional disorders and hypoglycemia (low blood sugar). After being introduced on the Merv Griffin Show as a "leading nutritional consultant," Fredericks was asked to estimate the number of Americans suffering from hypoglycemia. His reply, "20 million," has no basis in fact. Hypoglycemia is very rare. Several years ago, each of the past-presidents of the American Diabetes Association was asked to estimate how many patients he had seen with blood sugar disorders. All replies were similar: thousands of patients with diabetes (high blood sugar), but *almost none* with functional hypoglycemia.

Fredericks has written a column for *Prevention* magazine for many years. In 1976, *Prevention* invested $100,000 to sponsor a series of half-hour radio programs distributed free-of-charge to stations throughout the United States. According to Robert Franklin, the show's producer, Fredericks was paid $25,000 for taping the series. The programs generated large numbers of letters from desperately ill people, many of whom seemed to think that Fredericks was a medical doctor. (This is not surprising because generally he is introduced simply as "Dr. Fredericks.") Franklin was so disillusioned by the mail that he decided to syndicate a program which gave *reputable* advice, and the Harvard University School of Public Health agreed to sponsor it for three years.

Fredericks' books sell at handsome royalties. All of them attack the medical profession, cite questionable advice, and attribute therapeutic qualities to foods and food supplements. In person, Fredericks is charming and persuasive. He uses humor to illustrate his points and to ridicule those with whom he disagrees. Overall, he encourages unsafe degrees of self-diagnosis and self-treatment.

New Strategy

In 1961, the FDA dismantled what was probably the largest organized health scam up to that time—the promotion of "Nutri-Bio" by more than 75,000 full and part-time sales agents. Directly and indirectly, the product was being recommended as the answer to practically all health problems. Company literature containing misleading claims also included the book, *Stay Young and Vital*, by Hollywood actor Bob Cummings, a Nutri-Bio vice president. Huge quantities of other sales literature were involved in the case. In the Chicago area alone, Nutri-Bio agents turned in close to 50 tons of it for destruction.

The prosecutions of Nutri-Bio, Foods Plus, Lelord Kordel and Adolphus Hohensee were part of a vigorous FDA campaign in the late 1950s and early 1960s. During this period, more than 200 successful actions for misbranding were carried out, several prominent faddists were sentenced to prison, and the courts ruled that *any* false message given *in the context of a sale* could be considered part of a product's labeling. The 1962 Kefauver-Harris Amendment to the Food, Drug and Cosmetic Act, which made it illegal to market a drug until it is proven effective, added still another weapon against quackery.

By 1965, it must have been clear to leaders of the health food industry that marketing products labeled with false claims was a risky business. But the industry soon reorganized to get around the law. Most food supplement manufacturers stopped having their products falsely labeled as effective against specific diseases. Industry emphasis shifted somewhat from "miracle" drugs to "nutritional insurance," an approach which tends to attract little attention from federal prosecutors. "Specialization" developed whereby most publicists of misleading nutritional claims would no longer have direct financial ties to the sale of specific products. And common substances—vitamins, minerals, herbs and the like—would be promoted through the media without reference to brand names.

Thus, instead of claiming that his vitamin X preparation would cure cancer or flat feet, a manufacturer could rely upon books, magazine articles and talk shows to publicize the supposed benefits of vitamin X or the supposed difficulty of getting enough of it in one's diet. *In effect, the media became the label!*

By the mid-1960s, the health food industry was well-established, but had not yet captured the average person's mind. Most of its customers were considered cultists. Two developments changed this, however. The first was the explosive growth of mass communication, particularly television. The second was the growing public concern about pollution. Rachel Carson's *Silent Spring*, though filled with errors, increased public concern about pesticides and decreased public confidence in government protection. "Organic farming" promoters became able to arouse the interest of many people who weren't looking for magic, but just wanted to feel safer. Sales pitches like "Make sure you have enough!," "Beware of chemicals in our food!" and "Buy natural!" converted the majority of Americans into at least occasional customers.

The High Priestess

At the 1969 White House Conference on Food and Nutrition, the panel on deception and misinformation agreed that Adelle Davis was probably the most damaging source of false nutrition information in the nation. She promoted hundreds of nutritional tidbits and theories, many of which were unfounded. She stated incorrectly that fertile eggs were better than infertile eggs, and that crib deaths could be prevented by breast feeding plus vitamin E. Most of her ideas were harmless unless carried to extremes, but some were very dangerous. She suggested magnesium as a treatment for epilepsy, and she recommended dangerously high doses of vitamins A and D.

In 1971, a 4-year-old victim of Adelle Davis' advice was hospitalized at the University of California Medical Center in San Francisco. The child appeared pale and chronically ill. She was having diarrhea, vomiting, fever and loss of hair. Her liver and spleen were enlarged, and other signs suggested she had a brain tumor. Her mother, "a food faddist who read Adelle Davis religiously," had been giving her large doses of vitamins A and D plus calcium lactate. Fortunately, when these supplements were stopped, the little girl's condition improved. Two other young victims of Ms. Davis' advice—one crippled, the other killed—are described in Chapter 12.

Ms. Davis was the first "health authority" among modern food faddists who had any formal professional background. She was trained in dietetics and nutrition at the University of California at Berkeley, and got an M.S. degree in biochemistry from the University of Southern California in 1938. Many of her former classmates and teachers have affectionate memories of her past promise and were greatly distressed by her subsequent activities. Her books, which are full of inaccuracies, are not on the approved list of any responsible nutrition society.

Let's Eat Right to Keep Fit was Ms. Davis' most popular book. Professor George Mann of Vanderbilt University School of Medicine undertook the fatiguing task of documenting the book's errors and found an average of one mistake per page. Some of the errors are dangerous. For example, the suggestion that certain patients with kidney disease should take potassium chloride is one which could prove fatal.

In *Let's Get Well*, Ms. Davis listed 2,402 references to "document" its 34 chapters. Readers may well be impressed with this enormous list, but many of these references don't back up what she says in the book. For example, 27 out of the 57 references listed in Chapter 12 contain no data to support what she says in the chapter. A reference given in her discussion of "lip problems" and vitamins turns out to be an article about influenza, apoplexy and aviation, with mention of neither lips nor vitamins. Dr. Victor

Herbert has noted that in each instance where she referred to a scientific paper written by him, she misrepresented what he wrote.

In April 1972, a group of distinguished nutritionists had an opportunity to ask Ms. Davis to indicate what scientific evidence backed up many of her speculations. Like most food faddists, she did not base her ideas on such evidence. To question after question, she answered, "I will accept your criticism," "I could be wrong" or "I'm not saying it does." But she never told her followers that many of her claims had no factual basis or could be harmful.

Adelle Davis used to say that she never saw anyone get cancer who drank a quart of milk daily, as she did. She stopped saying that when she died of cancer in 1974, leaving behind her a trail of 10 million books sold and a large and devoted following.

The Chemist

Publication in 1970 of the book, *Vitamin C and the Common Cold,* by Linus Pauling, turned millions more people onto vitamins. Throughout the book, Pauling is convinced that large doses of vitamin C can prevent colds and decrease their severity. He states that daily intake of 200 milligrams (mg) will decrease the incidence of colds by about 15 percent, and that daily intake of 1,000 mg will decrease colds by 45 percent. (The Recommended Dietary Allowance of vitamin C is 60 mg.) Pauling bases his beliefs on his interpretations of experiments by others plus his own personal experiences. Looking at the same data, however, almost all medical and nutrition experts disagree with him.

Scientific fact is established when the same experiment is carried out over and over again with the same results. To test the effect of vitamin C on colds, it is necessary to compare groups which get the vitamin to similar groups which get a placebo (a dummy pill which looks like the real thing). Only in this way is it possible to determine whether the effect of vitamin C is greater than the effect of doing nothing. Since the common cold is a very variable illness, proper tests must involve hundreds of people for significantly long periods of time.

Largely because of Pauling's prestige, test after test has been carried out to determine whether vitamin C is of value in the treatment of the common cold. After considering the evidence, most medical scientists conclude that large doses of vitamin C do not prevent colds or shorten their duration. Vitamin C may have a small, antihistamine-like effect on the severity of cold symptoms, but large doses can cause a variety of medical problems (described in Chapter 1).

Pauling has also been recommending massive doses of vitamins for the treatment of severe mental illness. The vast majority of pyschiatrists reject this idea; and an American Psychiatric Association task force which reviewed the evidence several years ago found it entirely lacking in credibility. Recently, Pauling has been advocating megadoses of vitamin C for the prevention and treatment of cancer. In an interview in the July 1979 issue of *Prevention*, he estimates that the incidence and death rate from cancer "could be decreased 75 percent by the proper use of vitamin C alone." But a study at the Mayo Clinic, published in the *New England Journal of Medicine* in 1979, found vitamin C worthless for the treatment of cancer.

The Linus Pauling Institute of Medicine, founded in 1973, is dedicated to "orthomolecular medicine." This is based on the speculation that varying (usually by raising) the concentrations of substances (such as vitamins) normally present in the human body may improve health and help to prevent or treat various diseases. Here, too, Pauling's prestige is helping to elevate megavitamins from mere flim-flam to a controversial issue.

The relationships between Pauling and other promoters of vitamins are noteworthy. In a little-publicized chapter of *Vitamin C and the Common Cold*, Pauling attacks the health food industry for misleading its customers. Pointing out that "synthetic" vitamin C is identical with "natural" vitamin C, he warns that higher priced "natural" products are a "waste of money." And he adds that "the words 'organically grown' are essentially meaningless— just part of the jargon used by health food promoters in making their excess profits, often from elderly people with low incomes."

Despite these criticisms, Pauling was welcomed with open arms by the health food industry and participated in its campaign for legislation to weaken FDA protection of consumers against misleading nutrition claims (see Chapter 10). The largest corporate donor ($100,000 a year) to his Institute is Hoffmann-La Roche, the pharmaceutical giant which is the dominant factor in worldwide production of vitamin C. Many of the Institute's individual donors have been solicited with the help of Rodale Press (publishers of *Prevention* magazine) and related organizations which publicized the Institute and allowed the use of their mailing lists. Curiously, the 1976 edition of Pauling's book, retitled *Vitamin C, the Common Cold and the Flu*, contains no criticisms of the health food industry, its "jargon" and its "excess profits."

This omission was not accidental. After his first book came out, Pauling recently informed Dr. Barrett, he was "strongly attacked by people who were also attacking the health food people." His critics were so "biased," he decided, that he would no longer help them attack the health food industry while another part of their attack was directed at him.

In 1977 and 1979, Pauling received awards and presented his views on vitamin C at the annual conventions of the National Nutritional Foods Association. In 1981, he accepted an award from the National Health Federation for "services rendered in behalf of health freedom" and gave his daughter a life membership in this organization. NHF, as detailed in Chapter 10, promotes the gamut of quackery. Thirteen of its leaders have been in legal difficulty and five have even received prison sentences for questionable "health" activities. Pauling has also appeared as a speaker at a Parker School for Professional Success Seminar, a meeting where chiropractors are taught highly questionable methods of building their practices. An ad for the meeting invited chiropractors to pose with Dr. Pauling for a photograph (which presumably could be used for publicity when the chiropractors returned home).

Although Pauling's megavitamin claims lack the evidence needed for acceptance by the scientific community, they have been accepted by large numbers of people who lack the scientific expertise to evaluate them. After all, he's a distinguished Nobel Prize winner. And that's good enough for John Q. Public who assumes that a 1954 prize in chemistry means that subsequent claims in nutrition must be valid.

The Dentist

Like Linus Pauling, Emanuel Cheraskin is a professional who is trained in one area but speaks out frequently in another. A dentist, he has been promoting a wide variety of questionable nutrition ideas in papers for professionals and books for the general public. He and Carlton Fredericks also speak frequently at nutrition seminars for chiropractors.

In *New Hope for Incurable Diseases*, Dr. Cheraskin and a fellow dentist, W. M. Ringsdorf, Jr., make many wild claims. Thiamin in 2 mg doses will increase intelligence up to five times. Vitamin C will improve the behavior of schizophrenics. Carrot and lettuce juice make the hair shine. Liver juice helps diabetics, and spinach juice gives an extra boost of energy. The book also advocates treatment of glaucoma with vitamin C. Even harmless advice may be given for a senseless reason. For example, "Eat fresh fruits and vegetables to slow down aging." In 1972, Dr. C. E. Butterworth, Jr., director of the nutrition program at the University of Alabama (where Cheraskin and Ringsdorf were on the dental faculty), wrote a devastating review of the book, closing with:

> One expects more from university professors who write interpretations of science for the general public. This book has apparently been written for the faddist fringe and "health" food store market and for readers who seemingly *want* to believe in the miracles wrought by diet without regard for scientific evidence.
>
> Surely hope is an essential element of life, both to the sufferer from an incurable disease and the members of his family. But it is cruel to raise false hope under any pretense. In my opinion, this book raises nothing but false hopes, many of them not even new, in the mind of an uneducated reader.

In his latest book, *Psychodietetics*, Cheraskin admits that he has failed to convince most health professionals (who are qualified to evaluate his claims) and thus takes his case to the general public where he expects "a more enthusiastic response."

The Clinicians

Evan Shute, who died in 1978, was a physician in the business of treating patients. His primary interest was in vitamin E. Since this vitamin was synthesized in 1938, physicians as well as laymen have tried using it for many ailments. In 1946, worldwide interest was aroused by a report from Dr. Shute (an obstetrician and gynecologist), his brother Wilfred (a heart specialist), and Dr. Albert Vogelsang. The three Canadians claimed that large doses of vitamin E were beneficial in four major types of heart disease. But these claims could not be confirmed by other groups throughout the world.

Evan Shute's book, *The Heart and Vitamin E and Related Matters*, recommends vitamin E for the prevention and treatment of high blood pressure, gangrene, nephritis (a kidney disease), angina pectoris, varicose veins and other conditions. The book also claims that vitamin E can heal wounds without scars and can prevent senility and stroke if taken from an early age.

The Shute Institute, founded in 1948, is located in London, Ontario. It is managed by the Shute Foundation for Medical Research, which is supported by fees, gifts and bequests. Evan Shute remained at the Shute Institute, while Wilfred Shute entered private medical practice in Vancouver, British Columbia, in 1957.

In 1949, the Institute began publication of *The Summary*, its "scientific journal." The prime reason for publication of *The Summary*, admitted Evan Shute, "was the inability of the Shute Foundation to get its presentations published in North American medical journals." That should tell us something. Reputable scientific journals accept only papers in which warranted conclusions are drawn from adequate, well-designed experiments—such as those which compare treated and untreated groups. But Evan Shute's ideas were *not* based upon such studies. In fact, he regarded them as "unethical, illegal and immoral."

The Salesmen

Man has been a creature of fallacy ever since time began. It seems to be inherent in his nature to believe in false things . . . In the field of medicine, especially, man seems to delight in being completely taken in.

J. I. Rodale, who wrote this in 1954, seemed to understand how gullible people can be. Like Carlton Fredericks, Rodale had changed his original name (Jerome Irving Cohen) to one that was more promotable. Rodale was a shrewd businessman. His financial success attracted considerable attention in the early 1970s, and the publicity he received boosted his profits even more. He died in 1971, leaving a publishing empire to his son Robert.

By 1980, Rodale Press had a reported gross income of $80 million a year. *Prevention*, its major magazine, had a circulation of 2.4 million; and the circulation of *Organic Gardening and Farming*, its number two publication, was over one million.

J. I. Rodale was best known for his interests in "organic farming" and "health foods." Most media accounts of his work regarded him as eccentric, but harmless. A few brief mentions of the unscientific nature of his health concepts appeared in AMA and FDA publications, but for the most part he was ignored by medical scientists. This is unfortunate because he did a great deal of harm.

Prevention magazine contains easy-to-read articles on a variety of health topics. A few articles contain practical health tips, but most articles are misleading. *Prevention*'s primary message is that *everyone* should supplement his diet with extra nutrients. To support this point of view, the magazine uses most of the sales tactics described in Chapter 2 of this book. Articles and editorials often give equal weight to valid and invalid research, good and poor reasoning, scientific fact and health nonsense. Readers are told that our food supply is depleted of nourishment. News of nutritional "discoveries" is slanted to suggest that people who take food supplements are likely to benefit from discoveries which are just around the corner. Each issue contains a full-length testimonial story (for which the magazine pays $300) and some two dozen letters from readers telling how nutritional remedies have supposedly helped them.

Flyers sent to prospective advertisers refer to Prevention as "a uniquely constructed and productive advertising medium." A typical issue of the magazine contains 60-80 pages of food supplement advertising which costs about $13,000 for black-and-white pages and $17,000 for color pages. It is official policy to accept no ads for "remedies and cures," and with rare exception, the ads make no health claims at all. The reason for these policies is obvious. If claims of the type found in the articles, editorials and testimonial letters next to the ads were placed in the ads, sellers could be prosecuted for fraud and misbranding. False claims in the magazine's text, however, are shielded by freedom of the press. A 1973 survey reported that families that subscribe to Prevention spent an average of $190 per year for vitamin supplements and health foods. Today that figure is probably much higher.

Prevention will accept ads for books that promote unproven methods—including cancer quackery. "Books are really not products, but ideas," explains the Advertising Committee. "And ideas, we strongly believe, should be accepted or rejected not by a communications medium . . . but by each individual on a personal basis. The First Amendment to the United State Constitution guarantees freedom of speech, and we are not about to abrogate that hard-won freedom at Rodale Press." Prevention also accepts ads for questionable health services, such as hair analysis and the bizarre nutritional services of Dr. William Kelley described in Chapter 6.

According to Natural Foods Merchandiser, the largest single advertiser in Prevention is Natural Sales Company, the mail-order branch of General Nutrition Corporation (GNC) of Pittsburgh. GNC, with 800 stores, is the nation's largest health food retail chain. Its gross sales in 1980 topped $200 million.

In England, where the law is not as strict, J. I. Rodale, Ltd., markets Natrodale brand food supplements with false claims. Among them: "Eating bone meal will prevent insect bites, will almost completely stop cavities and will lower the pulse when it is high," and "Desiccated liver enormously increases energy." The English edition of Prevention is smaller than the American version and contains no date of publication. New issues are not distributed until the previous ones are sold. According to a Rodale

Press official, the market for health magazines and food supplements has been less profitable in England: "People there have less money to waste than they do in America."

Rodale ideas are summarized into the "Prevention System for Better Health," a mixture of sense and nonsense. The sense includes avoiding smoking and excessive coffee, getting exercise regularly, and eating nutritious foods. The nonsense includes recommendations for supplementary nutrients which at best are a waste of money, and at worst can be harmful.

J. I. Rodale imagined many dangers lurking in our food supply. He accused sugar of "causing criminals," and blamed bread for colds, stomach irritation, bronchitis, pneumonia, conjunctivitis, rickets in children and steatorrhea in adults. He warned that coke drinkers will become sterile. Even roast beef, pickles, ice cream and bagels aroused his concern. An article in the *New York Times Magazine* reported that each day, J. I. took 70 food supplement tablets and would spend 10-20 minutes under a short-wave machine "to restore his body electricity." He would live to 100, he told the reporter, unless he was run down by "a sugar-crazed taxi driver." But a few weeks later, at age 72, he died of a heart attack while taping a TV interview for the Dick Cavett Show.

Some people who laugh at Rodale Press's silliness may think of its overall set-up as harmless. After all, they say, Rodale does encourage people to do certain things which can improve their health. But nutritional scientists who look closely at Rodale Press are not amused. Its books and magazines are a significant factor in the growing public confusion about nutrition. And its political activities have caused a great deal of harm.

Although water fluoridation is an extremely valuable and *real* way to use dietary supplementation to prevent disease (tooth decay), Rodale Press has never recommended it. Before the death of J. I. Rodale, most issues of *Prevention* contained vicious attacks on fluoridation in articles, editorials and letters to the editor. Communities around Rodale's headquarters in Emmaus, Pennsylvania, have been subjected to an even greater amount of anti-fluoridation propanganda. In 1961, for example, Rodale Press spent more than $10,000 on a scare campaign which defeated a fluoridation referendum in nearby Allentown.

J. I. Rodale vigorously promoted bone meal tablets as a tooth decay preventive even though scientific authorities know they are not effective. (Recently, some bone meal tablets have been found to be contaminated with poisonous heavy metals such as lead.) In 1971, the Lehigh Valley Committee Against Health Fraud made an interesting observation. Ads for bone meal tablets occupied more than $50,000 worth of advertising space in *Prevention* during 1970. In addition, advertisements for filters claimed to remove fluorides from water occupied many additional thousands of dollars of space.

Scientists are also disturbed about Rodale's grossly unfair criticisms of pesticides and other agricultural chemicals which are badly needed to prevent starvation in many parts of the world.

In late 1971, Robert Rodale began a syndicated newspaper column called *Organic Living* which promoted romantic ideas about "nature" with only an occasional hint that our diets are deficient. To promote use of the column, *Prevention* readers were urged to contact local newspaper editors. After a year, some 40 newspapers were using Rodale's column, but editorial interest did not last. "Editors stopped using it," according to a source inside Rodale Press, so Robert stopped writing it during 1975. But several other ventures that began under his leadership—particularly magazines which cater to the developing public interest in conservation and physical fitness—have sold quite well. Robert, incidentally, studied journalism in college, but did not graduate.

Since the death of J. I. Rodale in 1971, Rodale Press has been trying hard to improve its image. *Prevention* contains fewer of the more obviously ridiculous types of ideas which J. I. used to publish. Its articles are more subtle, with less direct suggestion that vitamins will cause miraculous states of health. Readers are still encouraged to supplement their diets with many nutrients, both as part of the Prevention System and by slanted articles. Anti-fluoridation articles are not being published, although occasional letters to the editor from antifluoridation groups have helped such groups to raise funds. Subtle or not, Rodale Press remains one of the nation's leading promoters of health misinformation.

A recent article by Walt Harrington, top investigative reporter for the *Allentown Call-Chronicle*, revealed that Mark Bricklin, *Prevention*'s executive editor, recognizes that fluoride prevents tooth decay. When asked why the magazine has not told this to its readers, Bricklin replied, "It would only confuse them." Nor have *Prevention* readers been told that the human body cannot distinguish between "natural" and synthetic vitamins—a fact admitted to Harrington by Marshall Ackerman, the magazine's publisher.

Harrington also surveyed four medical school professors whose views had been quoted in *Prevention*. All four indicated that although they themselves had been quoted accurately, *Prevention* slants its articles to promote unnecessary supplements. (The magazine does this by failing to include any adverse comments by the experts it interviews.) One of the quoted experts was Stanley N. Gershoff, Ph.D., director of the Tufts University Nutrition Institute. When asked by Harrington whether healthy people need to supplement their diets as *Prevention* recommends, he replied, "I think that is nonsense. I certainly don't do it myself."

Year after year, *Prevention* readers will waste hundreds of millions of dollars on vitamin supplements and health foods because they believe in Rodale nonsense. But innocent children who get toothaches or empty bellies—as a result of Rodale efforts against fluoridation and scientific agriculture—will not understand the source of their suffering.

Attacks on Additives

Many school-age children have been labeled as "hyperactive" or "hyperkinetic." In 1973, Benjamin Feingold, M.D., a pediatric allergist from California, proposed that salicylates, artificial colors and artificial flavors were causes of hyperactivity. To treat or prevent this condition, he suggested a diet that is free of these additives. He recommended further that the hyperactive child be included in the preparation of special foods and encouraged the family to participate in the dietary program. Since foods prepared from "scratch" are necessary at all meals, the Feingold program is both time-consuming and financially expensive.

Many parents who have followed Feingold's recommendations have reported improvement in their children's behavior. In fact, many families have banded together into Feingold Societies (cults?) to promote the dietary program. But carefully designed experiments have failed to support the idea that additives cause hyperactivity. Improvement, if any, appears related to changes in family dynamics such as paying more attention to the children.

Because the Feingold diet appears to do no physical harm, it might seem to be helpful therapy in some instances. However, the potential benefits must be weighed against the potential harm of falsely communicating to a child that his behavior is determined by what he eats rather than what he feels. We feel sorry for the youngster who announced on a recent Phil Donahue TV show that he had misbehaved because he had "slipped" off his diet and eaten a candy bar.

Lendon H. Smith, M.D., another pediatrician, claims that allergies, alcoholism, insomnia, hyperactivity in children, and a variety of other ailments are the result of enzyme disturbances which can be helped by dietary changes. He recommends a variety of food supplements and an avoidance of white sugar, white flour, pasteurized milk, and other foods that are not "natural." His books include *Feed Your Kids Right* and *Improving Your Child's Behavior Chemistry*.

According to a Donahue show executive, "Unlike other M.D.s, Smith presents well on the air and has a special rapport with parents. He's funny, interesting and makes people feel good about themselves and their children."

In *Improving Your Child's Behavior Chemistry*, Smith writes how "It is amazing how children's behavior can be turned around 180 degrees by a vitamin C and B injection. Overnight, they sleep better, begin to eat, and are cheerful, calm and cooperative the next day." (Hey, Doc! Maybe they don't want any more shots!)

In *Feed Your Kids Right*, Smith suggests that a daily dose of 15,000 to 30,000 units of vitamin A is "about right for most of us." He also recommends a stress "formula" which includes up to 10,000 mg of vitamin C and 50,000 units of vitamin A each day for a month. These dosages, of course, can be dangerous—particularly to children.

In 1973, the Oregon State Board of Medical Examiners ordered Smith to surrender his narcotics license and order forms and placed him on probation for 10 years. The order, dated October 18, 1973, indicates that during the previous year, Smith had prescribed medication that was "not necessary or medically indicated" for six adult patients, one diagnosed as hyperactive and the other five as heroin addicts.

In 1970, a team of "Nader's Raiders" led by attorney James Turner published *The Chemical Feast*, a blistering but unfounded attack on the FDA. Said the book: "The Food and Drug Administration will not acknowledge the relationship between deteriorating American health and the limited supply of safe and wholesome food." During the following year, three other Nader associates formed the Center for Science in the Public Interest (CSPI) to investigate and report on a variety of food and chemical issues.

Two stated goals of CSPI are to "improve the quality of the American diet through research and public education" and to "watchdog federal agencies that oversee food safety, trade and nutrition." For three years, it sponsored a National Food Day to call public attention to supposed food issues. What issues? A 1975 Food Day brochure claims that "Chemical farming methods create environmental havoc." A 1976 brochure states: "Every few months, it seems, another common food additive is found to be harmful . . . And agricultural chemicals have polluted everything from the nation's water supply to mother's milk."

CSPI's Nutrition Action Project, led by microbiologist Michael Jacobson, holds that "most Americans get their information about food from ads by the big food corporations, which are . . . more concerned with big profits than with good nutrition." Who does CSPI recommend? Its recently released "Nutritional Hall of Fame" includes Adelle Davis, Benjamin Feingold and the Rodales. It also includes Jean Mayer, Ph.D., former Harvard University nutrition professor who is now president of Tufts University. Dr. Mayer, once the most prominent member of CSPI's Food Day Advisory Board, became outraged by statements in the 1975 Food Day brochure and resigned from the Board in protest. "If you don't understand modern agriculture," he wrote to Jacobson, "just stay out of it and don't encourage people to believe that small organic farms are going to give us all the food we need for the world."

Dr. Jacobson and his associates differ from the traditional attackers of chemicals in that they do not stress magical ideas about food. They are not obviously outlandish and do not appear motivated by personal financial gain. But they do oversimplify, sensationalize, and undermine public confidence in the government and the food industry—which lends credibility to what the faddists have been saying all along.

In 1972, CSPI did an excellent study of fluoridation which came out as favorable. The study report was minimally publicized by CSPI and soon went out-of-print. When subsequently asked to help promote fluoridation, Jacobson replied that his fluoridation expert had left and that CSPI lacked the resources to continue work in this area. But we can't help wondering whether this group, like Linus Pauling, does not want to take public positions counter to those of the health food industry.

Unfortunately, many of our country's largest and most respected food companies have also jumped on the "back-to-nature" bandwagon. Today the words "natural" and "additive-free" appear on almost every type of edible product. Even beer and candy bars (the so-called "health bars") bear these magic words. The hottest category in the breakfast cereal market are those called "health" or "natural" cereals—descendants of John Harvey Kellogg's granola. Loaded with sugar and/or honey, these cereals promote tooth decay when eaten as a snack without milk. They are also relatively high in calories, with some providing as many as 140 per ounce (compared to the 90-100 calories per ounce in the ordinary prepared cereals).

A recent article in *Natural Foods Merchandiser* notes that General Mills is buying the 14 Good Earth "health food restaurants" and hopes to at least double their number during the next few years.

Food companies which exploit the growing public fear of additives are likely to make windfall profits. But they will also be ignoring their responsibility to the American public. An educational campaign aimed at promoting sound nutrition and exposing food faddism would be a much more commendable course of action.

Crusading Groups

Promoters of questionable health ideas often form organizations to multiply their effectiveness. New groups are being formed at an alarming rate. How can one tell which are reliable and which are not? There is no sure way, but Gilda Knight, Executive Officer of the American Society for Clinical Nutrition, lists five questions which can help to evaluate a group:

1. *Are its ideas inside the scientific mainstream?* Some groups actually admit they were formed because their leaders were rejected by other scientists or they couldn't get their findings published in established scientific journals. That is a classic sign of quackery.

2. *Who are its leaders and advisors?* The International Society for Fluoride Research sounds quite respectable, but it is actually an antifluoridation group. The International Academy of Preventive Medicine numbers among its leaders Carlton Fredericks, Linus Pauling, Lendon Smith and other promoters of questionable nutrition practices. The Center for Science in the Public Interest lists Benjamin Feingold and a Rodale Press editor among its advisors.

3. *What are its membership requirements?* Is scientific expertise required—or just a willingness to pay dues? An organization open to almost anyone may be perfectly respectable (like the American Association for the Advancement of Science), but don't let the fact that an individual belongs to it impress you.

4. *Does it promote a specific treatment?* Most such groups should be highly suspect. A century ago, valid new ideas were hard to evaluate and often were rejected by the medical community. But today, effective new treatments are quickly welcomed by scientific practitioners and do not need special groups to promote them. The Association for Chelation Therapy and various groups which promote questionable cancer therapies like laetrile,

fall into this category. So do the American Schizophrenia Association (which promotes megavitamins) and its parent organization, the Huxley Institute for Biosocial Research.

5. *How is it financed?* The Nutritional Research Foundation was funded originally by profits from the notorious liquid protein diet of Robert Linn, D.O. The Council for Responsible Nutrition, despite its high-sounding name is a Washington, D.C., group that represents manufacturers and distributors of food supplements and other nutritional products. Don't assume, however, that funding by an industry makes an organization unreliable. The National Dairy Council and the Institute of Food Technologists are highly respected by scientific nutritionists for their accurate publications on nutrition.

All of us are exposed daily to many ideas about health, some of which are accurate and some not. Promoters of food faddism are working hard to gain your allegiance. When you are well, unless you are taken in to an extreme degree, what you believe may not matter much. But if you have a health problem—particularly a serious one—misplacing your trust can kill you.

Chapter 9

The Laetrile Story

Cancer quackery is as old as recorded history and probably has existed since cancer was recognized as a disease. Thousands of worthless folk remedies, diets, drugs, devices and procedures have been promoted for cancer management.

Laetrile heads the all-time list of quack cancer remedies. It is a trade-name for the chemical amygdalin, a substance abundant in the kernels of plants of the rosacea family, including apricots, peaches, bitter almonds and apple seeds. (These kernels taste bitter when their amygdalin content is high.) Such seeds are dangerous to eat because amygdalin is 6 percent cyanide by weight and releases cyanide when broken down within the stomach and intestine. Laetrile has been trade-named "vitamin B_{17}," but it is not a vitamin.

Amygdalin was first isolated by two French chemists in 1830 and has been listed as a cyanide-containing poison in the *Merck Index* since 1889. One-half gram of laetrile taken by mouth twice a day will produce significant blood levels of both cyanide and thiocyanate (a lesser poison). This dosage is often exceeded by laetrile practitioners!

Although amygdalin has been used against cancer for many years, there is no evidence that it is effective. In 1953, the California Medical Society published information on 44 cancer patients treated with laetrile during the previous year. Nineteen had died of their disease and there was no evidence that laetrile had helped any of the others. Laetrile's backers have not been able to show that it can control cancer in animals or humans. Many experiments at independent laboratories have also been negative. Without such proof, it is not legal to market the drug in interstate commerce.

Despite these facts, trafficking in laetrile has become big business. An estimated 50,000 to 70,000 Americans are using it each year. The cost of treatment varies with the methods used, the dosages of the drug and accompanying dietary supplements, and the cost of transportation and fees involved in visiting the doctor. A typical patient will spend thousands of dollars for a few weeks' initial treatment, followed by additional thousands of dollars per year for maintenance medication.

As often happens with quack remedies, claims for laetrile's effectiveness keep shifting. (That way when a particular claim is shown to be untrue, proponents can deny that it represents their current thinking.) Laetrile was first claimed to prevent and cure cancer. Then it was claimed not to "cure" but to "control" cancer while giving patients an increased feeling of well being. More recently, it has been claimed to be effective, not by itself, but as one component of "metabolic therapy," a program (with shifting components) that may include megadoses of vitamins, "pangamic acid" (also referred to as "vitamin B_{15}"), oral enzymes, coffee enemas, and a diet which excludes protein from animal sources. Two deaths from coffee enemas prescribed by naturopaths were recently reported in the *Journal of the American Medical Association*.

In July 1980, in response to political pressure, the Mayo Clinic and three other major cancer centers began a test of laetrile and "metabolic therapy" under the direction of the National Cancer Institute. The study included cancer patients for whom no other treatment had been effective, or for whom no proven treatment is known. All patients had tumor masses which could easily be measured, but most of the patients were in good condition. Half of the core group of 156 patients died within five months and only 20 percent were alive eight months after the study began. Since this is the expected result for patients receiving no treatment at all, laetrile and "metabolic therapy" flunked the test. Equally significant, cyanide toxicity occurred in some of the patients despite safeguards not used by "laetrile doctors."

The fundamental problem with laetrile chemotherapy is not that laetrile can't kill cancer cells, but that the dose needed to destroy a cancer also will kill the patient. When laetrile is dripped into two test tubes, one containing normal human cells and the other containing human cancer cells, the normal cells die as soon as, or sooner than, the cancer cells. Responsible physicians only use chemotherapy when the dose that kills the cancer is *less* than the dose that kills the patient.

Individuals Promoting Laetrile

Laetrile is one of several questionable remedies promoted by the late Ernst T. Krebs, Sr., M.D., of San Francisco. In the early 1920s, his Syrup Leptinol was seized by the FDA on charges that claims for it were "false and fraudulent." The syrup was sold at a time when the 1918 influenza epidemic was fresh in the public's mind. Its main ingredient was an herb which Krebs claimed had protected an Indian tribe from the "flu." He also claimed that his syrup was good for asthma, whooping cough, tuberculosis and pneumonia. Later Krebs promoted a supposed cancer drug called Mutagen, which contained the enzyme chymotrypsin. After that came laetrile—made from apricot pits during an attempt by Krebs to improve the flavor of bootleg whiskey.

The first federal action against laetrile occurred in 1960 when an interstate shipment was seized at the former Hoxsey Clinic in Dallas, Texas. Dr. Krebs and his son Ernst T. Krebs, Jr., then set up business as the John Beard Memorial Foundation. In 1961, in the second FDA action involving laetrile, the Krebs' and their foundation were also charged with shipping "pangamic acid" with claims that it is effective as a heart stimulant for humans and a tonic for race horses. Krebs, Jr., and the foundation pleaded guilty to five counts of violating the "new drug" provisions of the Food, Drug and Cosmetic Act. They were fined a total of $3,755 and Krebs, Jr., was put on probation for three years.

In 1965, the elder Krebs pleaded "no contest" to criminal contempt charges for disobeying a regulatory order prohibiting interstate shipment of laetrile. In 1966, he pleaded guilty to another contempt charge and was also convicted of failing to register as a drug manufacturer. The elder Krebs died in 1970 at the age of 95. In 1974, Ernst, Jr., and his brother Byron were each fined $500 and placed on probation for violating California's health and safety laws. Byron's osteopathic license was revoked later that year for "mental incompetence." In 1977, Ernst, Jr., was found guilty of violating his probation. When the appeals process ends, he may spend a few months in jail. Do you believe that would be sufficient penalty for year after year of serious lawbreaking?

Ernst, Jr., who is often referred to as "Dr. Krebs," considers himself a biochemist and a nutritionist. However, investigators have found that:

1. He was expelled from Hahnemann Medical School during the 1930's after failing his sophomore year.
2. He received an A.B. degree from the University of Illinois in 1942 after taking courses at five different colleges. He received low or failing grades in some of his scientific subjects.
3. His "Doctor of Science" degree is an honorary one awarded in 1973 by American Christian College, a small,

unaccredited and now defunct bible college in Tulsa, Oklahoma. The school, founded by evangelist Billy James Hargis, had no science department and lacked authority from Oklahoma to grant any doctoral degrees. Krebs received the degree when he gave a 1-hour lecture on laetrile.

Other Laetrile Promoters

The leading dispenser of laetrile is Ernesto Contreras, a licensed physician in Tijuana, Mexico, who considers his clinic "an oasis of hope," According to a recent advertisement, it is "one of the world's leading clinics in the prevention, early detection and Metabolic treatment of cancer, with more than 16 YEARS OF EXPERIENCE in more than 26,000 cases."

With all of this EXPERIENCE, you would think that if laetrile really works, Dr. Contreras would have little trouble assembling a series of his most impressive case histories for expert review. But several years ago, when invited to do so by the FDA, he submitted only twelve. Three of the patients could not be located. Six of the rest had died of cancer, and the other two had used conventional cancer therapy (making it impossible to judge whether laetrile had helped them). Are you impressed?

John Richardson, M.D., a general practitioner who operated a clinic in Albany, California, has also treated thousands of patients with laetrile. His license was revoked in 1976 by the Board of Medical Quality Assurance, which characterized his treatment of cancer patients as "an extreme departure from the standard practice of medicine" in connection with the deaths of several patients to whom he gave laetrile.

Laetrile Case Histories is a book by Dr. Richardson and his clinic nurse, Patricia Griffin, wife of another long-time laetrile promoter. John W. Yarbro, M.D., a prominent cancer specialist at the University of Missouri School of Medicine, has analyzed the book in detail. Although its cover promises 90 case histories, actual count reveals only 62. Dr. Yarbro concluded:

> The natural history of cancer in human beings is such that any large number of cancer patients contains a small percent with an unusually favorable clinical course. Thus, if Dr. Richardson selected his best patients, he could present a group with a survival time [much] greater than normal, even if no effective therapy at all were given. Even so, the patients

in his cases appear to have a survival time no better than would be expected on the basis of the natural history of cancer.

The Richardson Center, now located in Reno, Nevada, asks new patients to sign an elaborate disclaimer which states, in part, that:

My services in your case will be limited entirely, unless otherwise agreed, to nutritional consultation and nutritional therapy . . . I will not concern myself with the diagnosis, treatment, alleviation or cure of any specific disease process . . .

The Center's "nutritional" program routine includes "numerous vitamins, minerals, enzymes, and sometimes hormones or related medications." Its estimated cost for the first four months is $2,500 to $3,000, and a $2,000 deposit is requested during the first visit. The new patient agreement states that "laetrile is not a cure for cancer," but indicates that it is one of the "nutritional ingredients" which may be used.

Organizations Promoting Laetrile

The International Association of Cancer Victims and Friends (IACVF) was formed in 1963 to "restore the cancer victim's life and free choice of treatment and doctor." The Association's founder, Cecile Pollack Hoffman, was a San Diego schoolteacher who underwent a radical mastectomy for breast cancer in 1959. In 1962, she had further surgery due to the spread of the cancer. Her husband, while sitting in an airport waiting room, happened to pick up a paperback book entitled Laetrile: Control of Cancer, by Glenn Kittler, a leading laetrile propagandist.

After reading the book, Mrs. Hoffman sought further information. Not long afterward, she became a staunch supporter of laetrile and believed it had saved her life. Although she died of metastatic cancer in 1969, her organization has continued to operate. By 1979, it had about 50 chapters and 20,000 members.

IACVF sponsors conventions at which questionable cancer remedies are promoted and sometimes sold. It distributes information on the availability of these remedies and makes arrangements for travel to Mexico for treatment. IACVF members, who pay dues according to membership category, receive the Cancer News Journal which contains many misleading articles about questionable cancer treatments. Dr. Contreras is a "life member" of IACVF.

The Cancer Control Society was formed in 1973 in Los Angeles by dissident members of the IACVF after disputes over major policy and the distribution of the proceeds of book sales. The newer group favors aggressive lobbying and court action against government restrictions on questionable remedies of every kind.

The Committee for Freedom of Choice in Cancer Therapy, Inc. (CFCCT) was founded in 1972 by Robert Bradford, a former laboratory technician at Stanford University. This group was able to establish large numbers of local chapters throughout the United States within a matter of months. Some bookshops associated with the John Birch Society have served as meeting places for the Committee and as sources of literature about questionable treatments. The Committee has made wide distribution of a one-hour film called *World Without Cancer* as well as a book with the same name. Both products promote laetrile with false claims.

In 1977, Bradford, Dr. Richardson, Frank Bowman (Richardson's business manager) and Frank Salaman (CFCCT's vice president) were convicted of conspiracy to smuggle laetrile into the U.S. Bradford was fined $40,000, Richardson, $20,000, and the others $10,000 each. Records in the case indicate that Bradford received $1.2 million for 700 shipments of laetrile and that Richardson banked more than $2.5 million during a 27-month period. In his book, Richardson claims that this figure is misleading because his overhead was high and some of his money, shifted from one bank account to another, had been counted more than once. But the book also mentions that he treated about 4,000 patients for about $2,500 each, which would come to $10 million.

Bradford is currently president of American Biologics, a California-based manufacturer and distributor of laetrile and other questionable products. This company advertises that it is "an international agent for professional and patient referral" to Plaza Santa Maria General Hospital, a Mexican facility which offers treatment with laetrile, gerovital, chelation, megavitamins, enzymes, DMSO and several other questionable modalities.

The Political Explosion

Beginning in 1975, a steady procession of court cases aroused unprecedented media interest in laetrile. Government prosecutions, efforts to rescue children from "metabolic therapy," and suits by "terminal" cancer patients frequently made headlines.

The first major court case was brought by Glen Rutherford, a seed salesman from Kansas who believes that laetrile has been keeping him alive. About 10 years ago, Rutherford developed cancer in a rectal polyp. Fearful of surgery, he consulted Dr. Contreras who treated him with laetrile, recommended a change of diet, and *cauterized (burned off) the polyp*. Although cauterization cures this type of cancer when it is localized in a polyp, Rutherford emerged from his experience claiming that laetrile had cured him. (According to an article in *People* magazine, he also began taking 111 pills a day, most of them vitamins.) In 1975, he filed a class action suit, supported by the laetrile industry, seeking the right for "terminal" cancer patients to import laetrile for personal use.

Promoters of laetrile, cleverly portraying themselves as "little guys" struggling against "big government," then launched a campaign to "legalize" laetrile. (The fact that laetrile is big business was not mentioned.) With publicity and public distrust of government working to their advantage, citizens organized by the Committee for Freedom of Choice in Cancer Therapy began to pressure state legislators to allow the sale of laetrile within their states. Federal legislation to exempt laetrile from "new drug" laws was also introduced—by Larry McDonald, a laetrile physician from Georgia who became a Congressman.

Supporters of laetrile argue that individuals should have the freedom to choose their treatment, particularly if they are fatally ill. This argument is not valid! What is needed is freedom of *informed* choice. The laws which ban questionable cancer remedies are needed to protect the public from *all* types of ineffective remedies. The supposed psychological benefits of worthless remedies in apparently hopeless cases are far outweighed by the possibility that such products will be used *instead* of effective treatment and the fact that some of them are toxic. It is not possible to be certain in advance who is terminal. Even if it were, *is there any reason why our society should allow people who make false claims to take financial advantage and possibly speed the deaths of desperate cancer patients who would believe such claims?*

The first judge who heard the Rutherford case apparently thought so, for he ruled that any patient certified as terminal by any physician may import a personal supply of laetrile. Many state legislatures also thought so as laws were quickly passed to permit the sale of laetrile within 21 states. But as higher courts ruled on the Rutherford case, and as opponents of the laetrile fraud became better organized, the tide began to turn. In June 1979, the U.S. Supreme Court rejected the argument that drugs offered to terminal patients should be exempted from FDA regulation.

Laetrile proponents hope that if enough states pass favorable legislation, Congress may be persuaded to exempt laetrile from federal regulation, but they have made little progress toward this goal since the Supreme Court decision. Legal or not, the peddling of cyanide as a cure for cancer can be expected to continue for a long time.

Chapter 10

The Unhealthy Alliance

From 1972 through 1976, Congress received more than a million letters urging it to *weaken* consumer protection in the field of health. Responding to this pressure, most Congressmen became sponsors of legislation which would do exactly that. This strange situation was the result of an intense health food industry campaign led by an organization called the National Health Federation (NHF).

Millions of Americans mistakenly fear that they are not getting enough nourishment in their food. Many also hope that nutritional gimmicks are the key to superior health. In 1972, after 10 years of study, the U.S. Food and Drug Administration (FDA) proposed a number of marketing rules to combat this public confusion. Under these rules, many of the misleading sales tactics used to promote food supplements would have been forbidden.

NHF responded immediately with an all-out campaign to weaken the FDA. Lawsuits were filed to block the new rules, and Congress was urged to lessen FDA jurisdiction over food supplements and the false claims which help to sell them.

NHF's Leaders

The reason for NHF involvement in this issue is apparent from the backgrounds of its leaders. Many of them write or publish books or other materials which support unscientific health theories and practices. Many sell questionable "health" products and some have even been convicted of crimes while engaged in this kind of activity.

• Fred J. Hart, NHF's founder, was president of the Electronic Medical Foundation for many years. In 1954, Hart and his foundation were ordered by a U.S. District Court to stop distributing 13 electrical devices with false claims that they could diagnose and treat hundreds of diseases and conditions. In 1962, Hart was fined by the court for violating this order. He died in 1976. His widow is NHF's executive vice president.

• Royal S. Lee, D.D.S., a nonpracticing dentist who died in 1967, helped Hart found NHF and served on its board of governors. Lee founded the Vitamin Products Company, which sold food supplements, and the Lee Foundation for Nutritional Research, a prolific distributor of literature on nutrition and health. One of the vitamin company's products was "Catalyn," a patent medicine that contained milk sugar, wheat starch, wheat bran and other plant material. During the early 1930s, a shipment of Catalyn was seized by the FDA and destroyed by court order because it was being marketed with false claims of effectiveness against a variety of serious diseases. In 1945, Lee and his company were ordered by the FDA to discontinue a number of claims for Catalyn and other products. In 1956, the Post Office Department charged Lee's foundation with fraudulent promotions of a book called *Diet Prevents Polio*. The foundation agreed to discontinue the challenged claims. In 1962, Lee and his Vitamin Products Company were convicted of misbranding 115 special dietary products by making false claims for the treatment of more than 500 diseases and conditions. Lee received a one-year suspended prison term and was fined $7,000.

• Kurt W. Donsbach, chairman of NHF's board of governors, is a chiropractor and naturopath by background who worked for Royal Lee as a "research associate" for several years. In 1970, while Donsbach operated a health food store, agents of the Fraud Division of the California Bureau of Food and Drug observed him representing that vitamins, minerals and herbal tea would control cancer, cure emphysema (a chronic lung disease) and the like. Charged with nine counts of such illegal activity, Donsbach pleaded guilty to one count of practicing medicine without a license and agreed to cease "nutritional consultation." Most of the products Donsbach was "prescribing" to his "patients" were packaged by Westpro Labs, a company which he owned and operated. He paid a fine and served two years' summary probation.

In 1973, Donsbach was charged with nine more counts of illegal activity, including misbranding of drugs; selling, holding for sale, or offering for sale, new drugs without having the proper applications on file; and manufacturing drugs without a license. After entering a plea of "no contest" to one of the "new drug" charges, he was ordered to pay a small fine and was placed on two years' summary probation with the provision that he rid himself of all proprietary interest in Westpro Labs.

Although he sold the company to RichLife, Inc., of Anaheim, California, Donsbach remained affiliated as an advisor and lecturer. In 1974, he was found guilty of violating his probation and was fined again. He then became president of Metabolic Products, a company specializing in "orthomolecular concepts," which he sold in 1975. According to literature from Metabolic Products, its garlic extract could "prevent cellular deterioration," its alfalfa product had "anti-toxin properties" which could help to overcome "-itis diseases," and so on. RichLife currently sells *Dr. Donsbach's Pak Vitamins,* 17 different "specialized formulas" to "help make your life less complicated, more healthy." Among the products are an *Arth Pak,* an *Athletic Pak,* a *Dynamite Pak,* a *Health and Beauty Pak* and a *Stress Formula Pak.*

• Victor Earl Irons, vice chairman of NHF's board of governors, received a one-year prison sentence in 1957 for misbranding "Vit-Ra-Tox," a vitamin mixture sold door-to-door. In 1959, shipments of eight products and accompanying literature shipped by V.E. Irons, Inc., were destroyed under a consent decree because the products were being promoted with false or misleading claims. Other seized products were ordered destroyed in 1959 and 1960. According to a 1978 brochure from the V. E. Irons Company, "the *most important* procedure toward regaining your Health is the COMPLETE and THOROUGH cleansing of the colon." The products necessary for its "Vit-Ra-Tox Seven Day Cleansing Program" could be purchased for $65.50

• Andrew S. Rosenberger has been listed as NHF "nutrition chairman" and has been a featured speaker at NHF conventions. For many years, he and his brother Henry operated a large chain of health food stores called Nature Food Centers. In 1938, their firm made an agreement with the FTC to stop making therapeutic claims for more than 20 products. During the 1950's, the Post Office Department filed a number of complaints against the firm for making false therapeutic claims for various products. In each case, the company agreed to discontinue the claims. In 1962, the Rosenberger brothers were fined $5,000 each and given 6-month suspended prison sentences for misbranding dietary products. Nature Food Centers was fined $10,000.

• Clinton Miller, NHF executive director and legislative advocate, had a quantity of "dried Swiss whey" seized from his Utah wheat shop in 1962. The FDA charged that the product was misbranded as effective in treating intestinal disorders. The whey was returned when Miller agreed to change its labeling. In 1976, he was an unsuccessful candidate for the U.S. Senate.

• Paul J. Virgin, NHF treasurer, is public relations director of the Alta Dena Dairy, a producer of raw (unpasteurized) milk. This dairy has been implicated several times as a source of *Salmonella* infection in raw milk consumers in California.

• Bruce Helvie, an NHF governor, had vitamin and mineral products seized by the FDA because they were marketed with false and misleading claims for the treatment of more than 25 diseases and conditions. The seized products were destroyed by consent decree in 1960.

• Roy F. Paxton, another NHF governor, headed a firm which sold an alleged remedy called "Millrue." It was distributed through agents and health food stores, as well as by mail through ads in an NHF publication. In addition, Paxton consulted personally with prospective customers, diagnosing them as having such diseases as cancer, arthritis and diabetes, and recommending Millrue for them. In 1958, Paxton and his company were fined a total of $1,200 for false and misleading labeling claims for Millrue. When they persisted in selling the product and promoting it through NHF's publication, the FDA again brought prosecution for misbranding. In 1963—the year that Paxton's term as NHF governor expired—he and his company were fined a total of $4,000 and he was sentenced to three years in prison.

• Bob Hoffman, another NHF governor, publishes two body-building magazines and sells bodybuilding equipment and food supplement products through his company, York Barbell Co., of York, Pa. In 1960, the company was charged with misbranding its "Energol Germ Oil Concentrate" because literature accompanying the oil claimed falsely that it could prevent or treat more than 120 diseases and conditions, including epilepsy, gallstones and arthritis. The material was destroyed by consent decree.

In 1961, 15 other York Barbell products were seized as misbranded. In 1968, a larger number of products came under attack by the government for similar reasons. In the consent decree that settled the 1968 case, Hoffman and York Barbell agreed to stop a long list of questionable health claims for their products. In 1972, the FDA seized a shipment of three types of York Barbell protein supplements, charging that they were misbranded with false and misleading bodybuilding claims. A few months later, the seized products were destroyed under a default decree. In 1974, the company was again charged with misbranding Energol Germ Oil Concentrate and protein supplements. The wheat germ oil had been claimed to be of special dietary value as a source of vigor and energy. A variety of bodybuilding claims had been made for the protein supplements. The seized products were destroyed under a consent decree.

Hoffman's current catalogue suggests that "If you are habitually tired, you may find that FATIGABAN can make a marked change in your life." (It contains desiccated liver, iron and B-vitamins.) The rest of Hoffman's many products are now sold without healing claims. In 1978, according to an article in *Health Foods Retailing*, he was president of 12 companies worth $25 million.

Despite his many brushes with the law, Hoffman has maintained considerable professional and social prominence. During his athletic career, first as an oarsman and then as a weightlifter, he received over 600 trophies, certificates and awards. He was the Olympic weightlifting coach for more than 30 years and has been a member of the President's Council on Physical Fitness and Sports. His 75th birthday was celebrated in Washington, D.C., at a large party whose participants included Senator Richard Schweiker (R-Pa.) and Jack Kelly, brother of Princess Grace of Monaco and former international president of the Amateur Athletic Union (AAU). According to the February 1974 *NHF Bulletin*, Mr. Kelly praised Hoffman's "inspiration to the many athletes of the world," President Nixon sent a "heartfelt message" of congratulations, and Senator Schweiker and his wife "set the tone of the party-spirit with a happy birthday song and cut the first slice of birthday cake."

Mr. Schweiker is now Secretary of Health and Human Services, the agency that oversees the activities of the FDA. Shortly after taking office, he posed for a congratulatory picture with Hoffman and NHF's Washington lobbyist. According to *Health Foods Retailing*, the health food industry has been "rejoicing" over Schweiker's appointment. He and Senator William Proxmire were the prime sponsors of the bill to weaken FDA jurisdiction over questionable food supplements!

• H. Ray Evers, M.D., another NHF governor, is a major promoter of "chemo-endartectomy therapy" (also called chelation therapy) for a wide range of chronic diseases, but primarily for coronary artery disease. He claims to have treated more than 15,000 patients since 1964. In 1976, at the FDA's request, a Louisiana federal judge prohibited Evers from using chelation therapy in Louisiana. Testimony in the case suggested that at least 14 patients had died from this therapy at Evers' hospital. Later that year, Evers was given a suspended prison sentence and two years' probation after pleading guilty to ". . . intimidating and impeding officers of the Internal Revenue Service." According to the IRS agents' report, Evers had cursed at them, threatened their lives, and attempted to run one of them down with his car when they visited his property in connection with a tax matter.

Evers then set up practice in Montgomery, Alabama, where,

despite FDA efforts, an Alabama judge allowed him to continue the use of chelation therapy. Patients admitted to Evers' clinic signed a doctor-patient agreement which reads in part:

> I understand that the type of therapy given at the RA-MAR CLINIC may not be in perfect agreement with the so-called orthodox methods of treatment as approved by the AMA, FDA, or HEW. I understand that the . . . therapy given here is the type that the Physician and I both agree is the correct future of medicine. (By the use of nutrition, enzymes, physical therapy, magnetic medicine, use of pyramids, etc., or any other modalities that may be used to benefit mankind) . . . I willingly request this type of therapy and will abide by the results.

In 1979, Evers moved his practice to the Bahamas. He left the U.S., says the January 1980 *NHF Bulletin*, because he was "tired of FDA harassment," he faced million-dollar lawsuits by survivors of two of his patients who died, and he was unable to obtain insurance coverage as a result of these various legal actions. Weekly rates at his 80-bed clinic ranged from $1,750 to $2,250 for non-cancer patients and from $2,250 to $2,750 for cancer patients! According to Jack Wilson, D.C., his chiropractic associate, Evers was unable to obtain necessary work permits from the Bahamian government and therefore set up practice again in Alabama in 1980.

• Emory Thurston, an NHF governor who died in 1981, was an active promoter of the worthless cancer remedy, laetrile. Pro-laetrile pamphlets edited by him were displayed at his booth at an NHF convention in 1973. When approached by an agent of the California Bureau of Food and Drug who told him she had cancer of the uterus, Thurston said he could supply her with laetrile. He instructed the agent to contact him at his office at the Institute for Nutritional Research in Hollywood. She did. During his next meeting, Thurston sold laetrile to the agent—*and advised her not to have surgery!* After additional evidence against Thurston was gathered, he was convicted, fined, and placed on probation for two years.

• James R. Privitera, Jr., M.D., another NHF governor, was convicted in 1975 and sentenced to six months in prison for conspiring to prescribe and distribute laetrile. In 1980, after the appeals process ended, he served 55 days in jail. Then, because he had been prescribing unapproved substances (including laetrile, calcium pangamate and DMSO) for the treatment of cancer, the California Board of Medical Quality Assurance suspended his medical license for four months and placed him on 10 years' probation under Board supervision. During the probationary period, Dr. Privitera is "prohibited from making any representation that he is able to cure cancer through nutrition." Nor may he even tell a patient he has cancer unless the diagnosis has been confirmed in writing by an appropriate board-certified specialist.

• Andrew R. L. McNaughton, another NHF governor, has been a central figure in the worldwide promotion of laetrile. In 1977, he was placed on two years' probation after pleading guilty to a criminal charge of conspiracy to facilitate the transportation of smuggled laetrile. He had a prior conviction in Canada for a stock fraud.

Others who serve, or who have recently served, on the 27-person NHF board of governors, include:

• Harald J. Taub, who was editor of *Let's Live* and *Prevention*, two magazines which strongly promote the use of food supplements.

• Norman J. Bassett, former publisher of *Let's Live*.

• David Ajay, president of the National Nutritional Foods Association (NNFA), a trade association representing some 2,500 health food retailers, distributors and producers. In 1978, Ajay announced "Operation Counterattack," a series of lawsuits against "detractors of our industry who have been calling us ripoffs" (see Chapter 11). NNFA maintains an active political program with a Washington attorney, Bernard Fensterwald, as legislative counsel. The organization files lawsuits and presents testimony to regulatory agencies and Congressional committees for the purpose of keeping government interference with the health food industry to a minimum.

During the past two years, NNFA has given gift packs of selected health food products to all members of Congress "to remind them of what the industry produces and stands for." It also maintains a political action fund to help favorable candidates, but according to attorney Fensterwald, the fund has never accumulated more than $5,000. Currently, he reports, NNFA is lobbying hard in Congress "to improve the school lunch program so that millions of young Americans will be exposed to health foods and good nutrition. In the long run, every NNFA member will benefit as the student body of today becomes the health food consumer of tomorrow." In 1980, when Congressman Fred Richmond (D-NY) noted "National Nutritional Foods Month" in the *Congressional Record*, the high cost of "health foods" was not mentioned.

- Max Huberman, past president of NNFA.
- John Hemauer, past-president of the National Association of Naturopathic Physicians, who died in 1976.
- L. P. DeWolf, who, according to NHF, has had "40 years experience in the organic produce field."
- Maureen Salaman, whose husband, Frank, was convicted in 1977 of conspiracy to smuggle laetrile into the United States.
- Bernard Jensen, D. C., a leading exponent of iridology, a system of diagnosis based upon examination of the eye.
- Ida Honorof, publisher of *"A Report to the Consumer,"* a twice-monthly newsletter which specializes in health topics.
- Floyd Weston, president of Health Research Institute, Inc. According to NHF, Mr. Weston organized a group of businessmen six years ago "to conduct a worldwide search for the answer to good health." One of his "discoveries" is an "electrodiagnosis" machine based on the theory that there is "an electric wiring system in the body—each organ having a wire that goes to a standard location in the hands and feet." According to Weston, the machine "verifies that exact condition of individual organs throughout the body. It differentiates between acute, chronic or degenerative stages and discovers these pathological processes when regular clinical diagnoses cannot detect them." Treatment is then administered with homeopathic remedies, vitamins and/or minerals.
- Robert S. Mendelsohn, M.D., author of the syndicated newspaper column, *The People's Doctor.* Although he has been chairman of the Illinois state licensing board, Dr. Mendelsohn considers himself a "medical heretic." One of his books charges that "Modern Medicine's treatments for disease are seldom effective, and they're often more dangerous than the diseases they're designed to treat"; that "around ninety percent of surgery is a waste of time, energy, money and life"; and that most hospitals are so loosely run that "murder is even a clear and present danger." Mendelsohn also states that chiropractors "can absolutely be trusted." In 1981, he became president of NHF.
- Betty Lee Morales, president of the Cancer Control Society, a group which promotes questionable cancer "remedies." She is also a publisher and is co-owner of Eden Ranch, a firm which sells *Betty Lee Morales Signature Brand* food supplements. Promotional material from Eden Ranch suggests that Americans who do not use food supplements run a significant risk of developing deficiency diseases. Among its many supplement products are *Lipotropic Plus,* to relieve "liver stress," and *Nia-Flex,* to relieve stiff joints.

Nutritional Consultation

In 1976, the Lehigh Valley Committee Against Health Fraud answered an ad in *Let's Live* magazine which offered information from Eden Ranch about its food supplements. The reply contained a 2-page health questionnaire which we returned, indicating that the writer, "age 61," was in good health except that:

> For several years I have had (on and off) pain and swelling in the joints of my fingers and toes. During the past few months, I have had attacks of blurred vision. Sometimes my eyes ache and I see halos around lights at night. Your suggestions would be most welcome.

The arthritis symptoms, while not specific, were compatible with a diagnosis of gout, the one form of arthritis that can sometimes benefit from a special diet. The eye symptoms were taken from a textbook description of glaucoma, a condition that could soon lead to blindness if not medically treated. Mrs Morales' reply contained a disclaimer that her advice was for:

> public education . . . and to assist individuals to cooperate with the doctors of their choice in building better health . . . In the event that the information is used without the supervision or approval of a doctor, that is prescribing for yourself, which is your constitutional right, but we assume no responsibility.

Her "highly personalized nutrition program" consisted of "detoxification" with a special diet and enemas, plus 15 different food supplements which could be purchased from Eden Ranch or a health food store. Based on an enclosed price list, the supplements would cost more than $40 per month. They are of no medically recognized benefit for either arthritis or visual difficulty. *There was no apparent recognition by Mrs. Morales that the writer's symptoms might be serious or require urgent medical attention.*

In 1978, NHF persuaded the California legislature to pass a law that allows any person to give nutritional advice so long as no attempt is made to diagnose, prevent or treat any disease.

Donsbach University

Kurt Donsbach, chairman of NHF's board of governors, is also president of Donsbach University, a correspondence school which offers "qualified students an opportunity to complete the specific requirements of the University in a substantially shortened time frame of study, with no classroom or mandatory attendance required." Tuition is $1,495 for a "bachelor of science" degree, $1,695 for a "master's" degree, $2,195 for a "Ph.D." and $3,795 for a 3-degree combination program, with a 20 percent discount for advance payment. Payment may be made by Visa or MasterCard. Up to 25 percent credit toward a degree is given for "life experiences" such as working in a health food store, selling food supplements or reading approved books. An iridology course costs $1,495.

Most of the "textbooks" required for the "basic curriculum" are books written for the general public by promoters of questionable nutrition practices, including Donsbach, Carlton Fredericks, Gary Null, Emanuel Cheraskin, Roger Williams, Lendon Smith, Robert Atkins and Carl Pfeiffer (proponent of questionable diagnostic tests and megavitamin therapy for severe mental problems). The on-campus faculty in 1979 had seven members, including Donsbach, Ray Yancy (an iridologist) and Alan H. Nittler, M.D. (who, according to NHF, "lost his medical license in 1975 because he utilized nutritional therapies"). The school's advisory board has 15 members, including Mrs. Morales, Bruce Halstead, M.D. (a promoter of laetrile and chelation therapy), and Richard Passwater (a major promoter of selenium supplements and "vitamin B_{15}"). The school's first catalogue, a 4-page flyer, listed courses in "Super Nutrition" as required for both the master and doctoral degrees. But a recent ad promises "the finest quality nutrition education available anywhere."

Donsbach began awarding degrees through Union University, an unaccredited school in Los Angeles which opened in 1974. In 1977, the university formed a Department of Nutrition—with "Kurt Donsbach, Ph.D., Sc.D., as Dean of the Department." RichLife, Inc., the company which sells "Dr. Donsbach" supplements, then offered "scholarships" to its retailers who wished to further their education.

Donsbach says his Ph.D. was issued by Union University. However, the school's current president told a National News Council investigator that, although he has seen a diploma on Donsbach's wall, the school has no record of him as a student. (Donsbach replied that one reason he left Union was no confidence in the school's record-keeping!)

In January 1979, Donsbach University became "authorized" by California to grant degrees. This status has nothing to do with academic recognition, however. All it requires is the filing of an affidavit which describes the school's program and asserts that it has at least $50,000 in assets. Section 94310(c) of the California

Education Code states that it is unlawful for an "authorized" institution to represent or imply by any means whatsoever that any state agency has made "any evaluation, recognition, accreditation, approval, or endorsement of the course of study or degree."

In 1979, Donsbach began publishing the *Journal of the International Academy of Nutritional Consultants,* with Dr. Alan Nittler as its editor. The first issue had a press run of about 25,000 copies, most of which were sent free-of-charge to chiropractors. The second issue explained that Academy members could be listed in a directory, that the Academy "will in no way encourage or tolerate the practice of medicine under the guise of nutritional consultation," and would establish a legal fund to protect its members from "undue and unfair harassment by bureaucracies or agencies." Regular membership in the academy, *open to anyone,* costs $12 per year and includes a subscription to its journal. "Professional membership," which costs $50 per year, includes a directory listing plus a "beautiful certificate for your office." Sustaining membership, which costs $150 a year, gives a 15 percent discount on advertising in the journal. Most of the 47 sustaining members have commercial interests in methods promoted by the journal.

In 1981, the journal was renamed *Health Express* and Donsbach took over as editor-in-chief. Plans were also announced to market it through health food stores and newsstands.

One of the journal's many ads is for nutritional cassette tapes, made by Kurt Donsbach, which may be obtained by writing to "Dr. Donsbach's Tapes" at the same address as his school. A retailer who recently responded to the ad was sent two price lists, not from the school, but from Health Education Products, a company apparently located nearby. One list is for Donsbach's "Health Library" (of books and booklets) and cassette tapes (which include *Happier Sex Life* and *Herbal Medicine*). The other is for food supplement formulas such as *Optimum Nutrition, High Q, Anti-Oxidant Formula, Stress Nutrition, Renew-F* and *Renew-M.*

In 1980, Donsbach University announced a new masters degree (M.B.A.) program in chiropractic business administration, directed by Dom La Forte, D.C., dean of the university's new "La Forte School for Professional Business Management." Tuition is $1,695. Dr. La Forte, a California chiropractor, has for three years headed a practice-building firm which guarantees to increase a chiropractor's income by at least $50,000 a year without requiring him to do "anything in any way unethical." Its fee for six weekend seminars plus one year of consultation was recently raised from

$5,000 to $6,000, but now includes "free tuition" at Donsbach University.

Chiropractic assistants "with at least an Associate of Arts (A.A.) degree and/or a combination of actual work experience and study" can obtain a bachelor of science degree with one year of study at Donsbach University's new "Clydesdale School for Chiropractic Para-Professionals." Its dean is Joyce Clydesdale, a former associate of Dr. La Forte.

So far, about 2,000 people have taken courses at Donsbach University. Whether the mail-order diplomas they obtain will do anything other than mislead the public or enrich Donsbach remains to be seen.

Accreditation?

Donsbach recently announced that his university is "accredited" by the National Accreditation Association (N.A.A.) of Riverdale, Maryland. But this agency, itself unrecognized by the U.S. Secretary of Education, the Council on Postsecondary Accreditation (1 Dupont Circle, N.W., Washington, DC 20036) or the California Department of Education, has no standing among educators. An official of the California Department of Education has warned Donsbach several times to avoid exaggerating or misrepresenting the significance of N.A.A. "accreditation."

N.A.A. was incorporated under Arizona law in September 1980 by Clarence Edwin Franklin, Jr. (a chiropractor), and Linda Anne Franklin of Thousand Oaks, California. The two of them plus Clarence E. Franklin, Sr., were the initial board of directors. N.A.A.'s aim, according to one brochure, is to "operate an association for the accreditation of correspondence schools . . . which maintain non-traditional modes of instruction, content, and methodology." The Association was composed initially of four schools—two of them high schools. Donsbach University and one other school became "accredited" a few months later.

According to another brochure, ". . . N.A.A. provides institutions throughout the world with a single source of national and international recognition." Its accreditation process requires submission of a lengthy Self Evaluation Report for which "long range planning is advisable, especially in large schools where report preparation can take up to six months or more." The report must be accompanied by copies of all courses offered by the school which are then reviewed by "highly qualified professionals . . . usually practitioners in their field or instructors in institutions of higher education."

N.A.A's 3-person Committee on Accreditation includes Dr. Franklin and Stan Simmons, Ph.D., whose doctoral degree was awarded by American National University, one of the original four schools. A 1-year "probationary" period is required before accreditation can be granted. But according to Dr. Franklin, this requirement was "waived" for the six current members.

On June 3, 1981, Dr. William Jarvis, President of the California Council Against Health Fraud, Inc., paid a brief visit to N.A.A's office in Riverdale, Maryland. Here is what he reported:

> The "office" is a telephone in the living room of the bottom floor of a 2-family building in a run-down neighborhood. N.A.A.'s executive director, Glenn Harold Larsen, lives there with his wife and three children. The brass plate on his front door contains only his name. He told me that N.A.A. membership costs $30 per month. About $100 of the organization's $180 monthly income pays his salary and the rest goes for operating costs.

> N.A.A. correspondence designates Glenn Larsen as holding a Ph.D. degree which, he told Dr. Jarvis, is from Sussex College of Technology in England. But when Jarvis telephoned the British Embassy, he was informed that this "school" and its diplomas are not considered valid.

A Competitor?

Another organization now operating in Los Angeles bears considerable resemblance to some of Donsbach's programs. The University of Natural Health Sciences now offers an "accredited" mail-order "Ph.D." for only $1,495. According to the school's bulletin, which we obtained by answering an ad in NHF's magazine, the university is "registered (accredited) by the Natural Medicine Council. In fact, the National Medicine Council is the only nutrition accrediting organization in America, and is recognized as a national nutrition accrediting organization by the University of Natural Health Sciences. This accreditation speaks well for us." (If we understand this setup correctly, the school and accrediting agency are two parts of the same organization which recognize each other.) Consistent with the school's policy of offering admission "regardless of race, color, nationality, location, income, working hours, and educational background," the school's admission application requests no information at all about previous education. According to the school's bulletin:

Doctor of Philosophy (Ph.D.) graduates are exceptionally well received. The opinions of educated nutritional science professionals with Ph.D.'s carry more than ordinary weight. People listen to them when serious opinions and decisions must be made . . .

The prestige of being a Ph.D. graduate of the University of National Health Sciences and the right to state the fact that you are a Ph.D. graduate on your business cards, letterheads, signs and advertisements is an award of distinction that can lead to a wealthy satisfying life.

The National Medicine Council is open to "any individual, college or university affiliated with or engaged in the nutrition science field and otherwise answering all of the objects and code of ethics" of the Council. "Regular" membership costs $10 per year, "professional" membership costs $50, and "sustaining" membership costs $150. Applicants for regular membership are asked only their name, address and telephone number. Professional applicants are asked to indicate their professional degree and whether they wish to be listed in the Council's Registry Book as a "Nutrition Consultant." All members receive a monthly newsletter plus "a beautiful certificate for your home or office."

How NHF is Organized

The National Health Federation is a membership organization with headquarters in Monrovia, California, and a legislative office in Washington, D.C. Its members pay from $12 per year for "regular" membership to a total sum of $1,000 or more for "perpetual" membership. Many of the larger donors have financial interests in the matters promoted by NHF.

Because of the extent of its political activities, NHF cannot qualify as a charitable organization, and contributions to it are not deductible for federal income tax purposes. However, NHF advertisements and letters of welcome to members have stated otherwise. In 1972, responding to a complaint by the Lehigh Valley Committee Against Health Fraud, the Internal Revenue Service ordered NHF to stop misrepresenting its tax status.

NHF members receive occasional mailings and a monthly 32-page magazine which until recently was called the *NHF Bulletin*. (It is now called *Public Scrutiny*.) Members are also invited to attend frequently-held conventions, most of which take place in the Western part of the U.S. Visitors to such meetings have noted that most participants are people of middle age and older who are preoccupied with their health. Many exhibit a rigidly suspicious outlook, fearing that government is thoroughly failing to protect them from "poisons" in their food and from exploitation by medical and drug industries. In November 1974, during a brief visit to a NHF convention in New York City, we noticed that many of its 34 exhibitors were making misleading sales claims for their products. Most blatant was the claim that a sea-water concentrate would prevent cancer. Other items for sale included pyramids to wear on your head to ward off disease and books telling how to cure cancer with laetrile.

According to the *National Health Federation Handbook,* sold for 10 cents, any two members can start a local chapter by adopting the NHF constitution and bylaws, naming temporary officers and receiving clearance from NHF headquarters. The handbook envisions a pyramidal national structure with local groups selecting a county board of directors, county boards selecting a state board of governors, and state boards selecting one delegate each to join the 27 at-large governors at the national level. This structure is mainly hypothetical, however, since the number of chapters has generally been fewer than 100. National membership, estimated from *Bulletin* circulation figures, averaged about 21,000 from 1974 to 1979. During the same period, NHF's annual budget rose from $345,000 to $914,660. In 1979, with help from Richard A. Viguerie (the fundraising expert who specializes in computerized mailings for ultraconservative organizations), NHF's membership rose to about 40,000.

For three years, beginning in 1977, NHF's Washington office was closed for economic reasons. During this period, attorney James Turner was listed in the *Bulletin* as NHF's "Washington Representative." Turner, a former "Nader's Raider," is principal author of *The Chemical Feast,* a book highly critical of the FDA (see Chapter 8). As Washington Representative, Turner did not lobby, but was paid a small retainer to keep NHF informed about pending government regulations, legislation and the like. His position was terminated in 1980 when NHF hired Gertrude Engel, an associate of NHF governor Bob Hoffman, as a lobbyist.

NHF's Philosophy

Since its formation in 1955, the steadfast purpose of NHF has been to promote what it calls "freedom of choice" by health consumers. As stated in each issue of its *Bulletin*:

NHF opposes monopoly and compulsion in things not related to health where the safety and welfare of others are not concerned. NHF does not oppose nor approve any specific health profession or their methods, but it does oppose the efforts of any one group to restrict the freedom of practice of qualified members of another profession, thus attempting to create a monopoly.

At first glance, this credo may seem harmless and somehow related to opposing unfair business competition. What NHF really means, however, is that proven methods of treatment should not be allowed to drive quackery out of the marketplace. Under this philosophy, anyone who has a product or "treatment" which he claims can help people's health should be allowed to sell it. Scientific proof that a particular method works should not be required. Unless a method causes immediate death or serious injury, our government should not interfere.

Put in its simplest terms, what NHF wants is for quackery to be made legal.

The Scope of NHF Activity

NHF's publications and convention programs make it clear that NHF promotes the gamut of questionable health methods and has little interest in medically acceptable types of treatment.

Nutritional fads, myths, and gimmicks are mentioned favorably by NHF publications and convention speakers. Worthless cancer treatments, particularly laetrile, are promoted in the same ways. *Bulletin* articles look with disfavor on such proven public health measures as pasteurization of milk, smallpox vaccination, polio vaccination and fluoridation of water. Use of nutritional supplements is encouraged by claims that processing depletes our food supply of its nutrients. Use of "natural" products is encouraged by exaggerated claims that our food supply is "poisoned." Chiropractic and naturopathy are regarded favorably. Books which promote questionable health concepts are reviewed favorably in the *Bulletin*. Underlying all these messages is the idea that anyone who opposes NHF ideas is part of a "conspiracy" of government, organized medicine and big business against the little consumer.

NHF files many lawsuits against government agencies and joins in the defense of many people prosecuted for selling questionable "health" products or services. It is also very active in the legislative arena. It worked hard to support chiropractic inclusions under Medicare and has been vigorously opposing federal subsidies to communities who want fluoridation.

To bolster the influence of its lobbyist, its publications and special mailings may include form letters and instructions to urge legislators and other government officials to support NHF positions. Letter-writing requests almost invariably distort the issues and contain underlying themes of persecution, discrimination and conspiracy. For example, to arouse support for the anti-FDA vitamin bill, NHF suggested that FDA regulations would drive up vitamin prices, "take away our vitamins," and even make it illegal to manufacture most of the supplements now available.

Crying, "Fight for your freedom to take vitamins!" NHF organized its members and allies into unprecedented political activity. Article after article urging support of the anti-FDA bill appeared in the *NHF Bulletin,* in *Prevention* and other health food industry magazines, and in chiropractic journals. Letter-writing kits were distributed by chiropractors, by health food stores and in special NHF mailings. At a Congressional hearing on this issue, several Congressmen reported that they received more mail about vitamins than about Watergate!

As the mail piled up, most Congressmen lost sight of why it was coming—that their constituents had become confused and frightened by health food industry propaganda. (It was not apparent at the time, even to the FDA, that a substantial number of letter-writers were not merely users of vitamins, but were also *sellers* who worked for such companies as Shaklee and Neo-Life.) In 1976, a modified form of NHF's anti-FDA vitamin bill was passed by Congress.

NHF has also been promoting a "Medical Freedom of Choice" bill. Federal laws now require that all drugs be proven both safe and effective before they are marketed. NHF's proposed bill, which would remove the efficacy requirement, would open the door to any supposed "remedy" that doesn't kill people on-the-spot.

In recent years, the prime sponsor of such legislation has been Representative Steven Symms (R-Idaho). According to columnist Jack Anderson, Symms has received thousands of dollars from the pharmaceutical industry in campaign contributions and speaking fees. During his successful campaign to unseat Senator Frank Church in 1980, Symms received $2,500 from the political action committee of Pfizer, Inc., $3,000 from Dart Industries' political action committee, and lesser amounts from American Cyanamid and other drug-related firms. Although Symms' views predated his support from these companies, it is noteworthy that legitimate drug companies would support a legislator who would open the floodgates to quack remedies!

In 1973, a New Jersey-based group called Citizens for Truth in

Nutrition (CTN) was organized by a 23-year-old college student named Sam Biser. Although apparently independent from NHF, it was led by many NHF activists. Its major activities included anti-FDA meetings, media appearances and lawsuits contesting the pending FDA food supplement regulations. The legal approach was unusual in that Biser urged CTN members to file identical suits in each of the 11 federal court districts, to claim pauper status if possible, and to fight against consolidation of the suits into one proceeding. These tactics were obviously calculated to tie up FDA legal resources.

Like NHF, CTN's promotional literature claimed falsely that its contributions were tax-deductible until it was ordered by the Internal Revenue Service to stop these claims. The organization no longer appears to be active, but Biser and his brother Loren publish *The Healthview Newsletter*, "the newsletter on health and nutrition which believes there are *NO* 'incurable' conditions." Issued 4-5 times a year, it features in-depth interviews with prominent promoters of questionable remedies as well as testimonial letters from readers who try them.

Promotion of Laetrile

In February 1978, NHF began publishing *Public Scrutiny* as a monthly 16-24-page newspaper whose primary focus was on laetrile and "metabolic therapy." Most of its original staff members were prominent promoters of laetrile, and three of its advisers had been convicted of laetrile-related crimes.

Because laetrile lacks FDA approval as a safe and effective drug, it is illegal to transport it across state lines. However, cancer patients certified by any physician as "terminal" may legally import a six-month supply for personal use. Each issue of *Public Scrutiny* contains a full-page ad from the Laetrile Information Center, a company near the Mexican border, which will arrange for legal importation. Mexican clinics and other sellers of laetrile are also listed regularly in *Public Scrutiny*.

NHF's library is organized as a separate corporation. Contributions to it, which were tax-deductible, have been used to purchase transcripts of court cases and to support research favorable to laetrile. Early in 1978, NHF used Richard A. Viguerie to send its members a fundraising letter and poll. The letter announced that "the NHF Memorial Library has just decided to make legalization of laetrile its No. 1 priority" and would "conduct a major effort to mobilize Congressional support against the outrageous ban on laetrile."

Regarding the poll, the letter promised:

> Your responses along with the responses of other selected members of the community will be tabulated and released to the national press, the United States Senate Health Subcommittee and each of your senators and congressmen.

Public Scrutiny published the results of the poll in an article headlined "Americans Want Freedom of Choice." Over 90 percent of those who returned their voting cards favored NHF's position on each of the four laetrile-related questions. Hardly surprising, since only NHF members voted.

Recently a bill to exempt laetrile from FDA jurisdiction was introduced by *Public Scrutiny*'s legislative advisor, physician-Congressman Larry McDonald (D-Ga.). A malpractice suit against him by survivors of a patient he treated with laetrile was settled in 1979 for $30,000. When McDonald's bill was introduced, NHF sent members another computerized fundraiser containing petitions to Congress.

After the Lehigh Valley Committee Against Health Fraud reported the nature of Viguerie's mailing on behalf of the NHF library, the Internal Revenue Service revoked the library's tax-deductible status. (An organization whose primary activity is political action cannot have tax-deductible status for its contributions.) NHF is appealing this decision. A 1979 Viguerie solicitation which claimed (incorrectly) that gifts to NHF itself are tax-deductible, apparently stimulated more legal troubles for NHF. According to the May/June newsletter of NHF governor Ida Honorof, this mailing involved illegal use of a bulk mailing permit. The newsletter also reported that NHF received letters from the attorneys general of four states, "threatening litigation because NHF had never filed as a fundraising organization as required by those state laws." Ms. Honorof, alleging financial irregularities within NHF as well, then resigned as NHF governor.

NHF furnishes support to many people involved in laetrile court cases. Appeals in *Public Scrutiny* raised more than $5,000 to help defend NHF governor James Privitera; and after he was convicted, NHF generated more than 10,000 form letters asking California governor Jerry Brown to pardon him. NHF also gave $5,000 toward the legal expenses of the parents of Chad Green, a 3-year-old boy with leukemia, and an NHF governor served as a lawyer for the parents.

Chad attracted nationwide attention when his family moved to Mexico in order to defy a Massachusetts court order that the boy receive proper therapy and stop getting laetrile. Chad's progress was followed closely in *Public Scrutiny*. Two pages in the October 1979 issue described how Chad was thriving, how his father was studying for a career as a "nutrition consultant," and how Chad's mother had stopped his chemotherapy without telling the Mexican clinic doctor. A few days after the newspaper was distributed, the boy died. Chad's parents continue to promote laetrile and claim that he died because he "lost the will to live." However, the autopsy showed recurrent leukemia, and cyanide was found in his liver and spleen. We believe Chad would be alive today were it not for the laetrile industry.

NHF also assisted the parents of Joey Hofbauer, an 8-year-old boy with Hodgkin's disease, a form of cancer usually curable in its early stages. In 1977, New York State authorities sought custody of Joey because his parents chose laetrile over effective treatment for the boy. With NHF attorney Kirkpatrick Dilling representing the parents, the court ruled that they were "concerned and loving" and "not neglectful" in rejecting orthodox treatment. After 18 months of laetrile and megavitamin treatment from Michael Schachter, M.D. (a New York psychiatrist who sometimes lectures at NHF conventions), Joey was moved to the Bahamas for another type of questionable treatment. He died in 1980 with lungs full of tumor. According to an article in *Penthouse* magazine, treatment at Schachter's clinic costs $3,000 to $5,000 for the first six months and $3,000 to $4,000 thereafter.

The "affidavit" system under which personal supplies of laetrile may be legally imported into the U.S. is the result of a 1977 ruling in the case brought against the FDA by Glen Rutherford (see Chapter 9). This ruling is being appealed by the FDA. Rutherford is now an NHF governor, Kirkpatrick Dilling is one of the two attorneys handling the case, and NHF is now paying the attorney fees.

NHF's Fight Against Fluoridation

Scientists know that if children get the proper amount of fluoride in their diet, they will get many fewer cavities in their teeth. Adjusting community drinking water to about one part fluoride to one million parts of water is a safe, simple and inexpensive way to accomplish this. Although NHF's leaders claim to be interested in preventing disease by "proper nutrition," they fight hard against water fluoridation.

Over the years, NHF has assembled a great many documents which it claims are "proof" that fluoridation is dangerous (which it is not). Close examination of these documents, however, shows that they contain reports of poorly designed "experiments," twisted accounts of actual events, statements by respected scientists taken out of context to change their meaning, misinterpreted statistics and other forms of faulty reasoning. Given enough publicity, however, these items can convince many communities that fluoridation is too risky. Many innocent children have NHF to thank for their toothaches!

In January 1972, NHF granted $16,000 for a fluoridation study to the Center for Science in the Public Interest (CSPI), a group led by former associates of Ralph Nader. To help raise this money, a special mailing was sent to NHF members:

> SPECIAL URGENT APPEAL-NHF is proud to announce that it has undertaken to underwrite $16,000.00 in costs for the CLINICALLY controlled investigation of the long-term effects of fluorides in the human. This test is being conducted by FRIENDS of indisputable, scientific reputation. With this information we will be armed by unassailable, up-to-date, scientific data to help defeat fluoridation! There is NO such study available in the world at this time and the costs are amazingly low. The Executive Committee committed us to this obligation in emergency session . . .

When CSPI learned about this fundraising message, it protested, stating that the study would be a scientific review of available knowledge and that its outcome was certainly not fixed against fluoridation. NHF apologized, claiming that the fundraiser had been mailed "without being cleared by appropriate officials" and contained "serious errors" about the nature of the study. NHF members were never told of these errors, however.

In August 1972, a preliminary draft of the CSPI study was released to activists on both sides of the fluoridation controversy. This was done so that its author could get suggestions and criticisms from knowledgeable individuals before he wrote his final report. The final report was issued at about the same time as the December 1972 *NHF Bulletin* went to press stating:

> A good many months ago, NHF voted a grant to the Center for Science in the Public Interest to underwrite an unbiased study of total fluoride consumption and its influence on health. This was done on the anticipation that such a study, never before undertaken by a scientific body, would put the fluoride controversy into proper perspective. That study is

nearing its completion. Two preliminary, interim reports have been issued. It begins to appear as if most of the contentions of NHF on this question will be validated in this unbiased study.

CSPI's final report, however, did not "validate most of NHF's contentions." Rather, it concluded that " . . . the known benefits of fluoridation far outweigh any risks which may be involved."

The favorable outcome of this study was never reported to NHF members. In private communications, however, NHF claimed first that the study was "never completed" and later that it was unacceptable because its author ignored too much antifluoridation "evidence." A Rodale Press editor even suggested that the author had been "intimidated" or "bought off." Thus, having invested $16,000 in an "unbiased" study by "FRIENDS of indisputable, scientific reputation," NHF ignored its conclusions!

Do you think it possible that the study's author was intimidated or bribed? What actually happened was quite simple. After officials of the Lehigh Valley Committee Against Health Fraud reviewed the preliminary draft, they presented the author with a detailed analysis which included three main suggestions:

1. He should consider rewording certain passages which, although they contained accurate conclusions, could easily be used out of context to make his study sound unfavorable to fluoridation.
2. Instead of stimulating unnecessary doubt with vague statements that "not enough is known" about certain issues, he should state exactly what future research he recommends.
3. To place the entire study in perspective, he should make a clear overall comparison between the known benefits of fluoridation and the "unknown risks" which he thought were worth investigating.

When the author followed these suggestions, the report became politically worthless to NHF.

In 1974, NHF announced that opposing fluoridation would be its number two priority and that a biochemist named John Yiamouyiannis had been hired to "break the back" of fluoridation. Yiamouyiannis soon began issuing reports based on misinterpreted government statistics, claiming that fluoridation causes cancer. He was joined in this effort by Dean Burk, a retired National Cancer Institute employee who is also a leading promoter of laetrile. In 1978, after an article in *Consumer Reports* criticized their work severely, Yiamouyiannis filed suit for libel. The suit was dismissed a few months later by a federal court judge. A 3-judge panel of the U.S. Court of Appeals subsequently upheld the dismissal, commenting that preparation of the *Consumer Reports* article "exemplifies the very highest order of responsible journalism." A further appeal to the U.S. Supreme Court was also unsuccessful.

In 1980, Yiamouyiannis had a falling out with other NHF officials, left NHF and founded the National Health Action Committee, an organization whose structure and scope of activity appear virtually identical to those of NHF. After *NHF Bulletin* editor Don Matchan resigned to join forces with Yiamouyiannis, NHF stopped publication of its *Bulletin* and began issuing *Public Scrutiny* in magazine format.

The Unique Alliance

NHF thus stands revealed. Its policies disregard medical science and proven public health measures. Its leaders promote questionable "health" methods, often at personal profit. Its followers, although confused about the issues in which they involve themselves, are active in the arena of politics. For most of them, nutrition is a religion, not a science.

NHF and its allies are well-organized and working hard. Its leaders probably hold sincere beliefs in their health methods. Its followers sincerely believe they can improve their health by following the methods of their leaders.

Sincere or not, NHF can be dangerous to your health!

Chapter 11

Nutrition and the Media

With the words "WONDER DRUG" stretched prominently across the front cover of its March 13, 1979 issue, *New York* magazine announced that "B-15 cures alcoholism, hepatitis, heart disease, allergies, diabetes, schizophrenia, glaucoma, keeps you young and purifies the very air you breathe. Maybe." Inside the magazine, a three-page story, *Will Vitamin B-15 Cure What Ails You?*, follows a similar pattern. A few sentences contain cautions from the FDA, but the bulk of the article heralds the claims of promoters and suggests that the FDA and big drug companies have an ulterior motive to keep B-15 off the market. Almost overnight, the magazine later reported, it became "impossible to find the vitamin on any dealer's shelf in the metropolitan area for a full week." The fact that "B-15" is neither a vitamin nor a nutrient was not made clear to the magazine's readers.

Publicity is obviously a major factor—if not *the* major factor—in the sale of food supplements. We have already noted how nutrition misinformation is spread by word-of-mouth and in health food industry publications. This chapter focuses on the roles of talk shows, news reports, and articles in general publications.

The Handling of News

Information that will attract a wide audience is considered "newsworthy." It may be new, startling, alarming or amusing; or it can have any other quality which an editor or producer believes will interest the particular audience toward which his efforts are directed. Magical claims about "nutrition" tend to be regarded as more newsworthy than the "unvarnished truths" of nutritional science. The people who make these claims are also regarded as newsworthy. According to *Health Foods Retailing*, Gayelord Hauser, Emanuel Cheraskin and other industry leaders generated more than 25 media productions and stories in connection with the 40th anniversary meeting of the National Nutritional Foods Association, held in Boston in 1978.

If you were a writer, would you try not to arouse false hopes in your readers? A few years ago, 20 editors and reporters from Eastern Pennsylvania newspapers completed a questionnaire designed by the Lehigh Valley Committee Against Health Fraud. One question was:

Dr. John Banks, President of the National Nutrition Research Association, is the speaker at the local women's club which you often cover. He claims that a certain nutrient has great healing powers not yet sufficiently appreciated by scientists. He does not seem to be far-fetched, but his ideas are completely new to you. Would you be more likely to report this as a straight news event or to evaluate his claims by seeking another opinion?

Fifteen out of 20 (75%) said they would report this as a straight news event. Seven out of those fifteen said that even if they consulted a physician who said the claims were utter nonsense, they would still report the event without including any criticism! When questioned further, they said that reporters of news events should report them as they happen, *without making judgements.* If critics of "Dr. Banks" (a fictitious name) want their say, they should create their own news events to get coverage.

"Non-judgmental" attitudes of this sort, which are common among reporters, help explain why the sensational claims of popular "nutrition" are expressed so frequently in the media. The foolishness of these claims does not usually make them *less* newsworthy, and may even make them *more* newsworthy!

Several other factors work against health scientists who try to educate the public through the media:

1. Time works to quackery's advantage. It is much easier to report a lie as a straight news event than it is to investigate it.
2. Some journalists who have been misled by false nutritional ideas cannot write accurate reports.
3. Most promoters of nutrition misinformation are regarded as "underdogs" in a struggle against the "establishment." As such, they tend to be treated much more sympathetically than we believe they deserve. Most editors insist that articles which attack false ideas be "balanced" so that the apparent "underdog" gets a "fair" hearing. Even science editors who know the health food industry is selling the public a bill of goods rarely feel a duty to issue effective public warnings.

4. Many more people are actively promoting nutrition misinformation than are actively opposing it. The sheer force of numbers works against the truth.
5. Publications which accept ads for food supplements may be unwilling to risk offense to their advertisers. A blatant example of this occurred last year when *Self* magazine published an article by a freelance writer listing money-saving tips from Dr. Barrett's consumer health textbook. A tip about vitamins was deleted from the writer's manuscript by the magazine's editors.
6. Many editors fear that attacks on nutritional quackery will stir up controversy from readers who regard nutrition as their religion. Worse yet, they may be afraid that attacking the credibility of a promoter will provoke a libel suit.

Unbalanced Talk Shows

When a newspaper or magazine publicizes a questionable nutrition claim, most editors are willing to restore "balance" by publishing a rebuttal letter which contains accurate information. However, most talk shows which reach huge audiences do not have equivalent policies.

During the early 1970's, Merv Griffin had many promoters of megavitamins as guests on his show, but rebuttal requests from qualified nutritionists were ignored. During the past five years, Phil Donahue has given tremendous publicity to the ideas of Benjamin Feingold, Lendon Smith and Robert Mendelsohn. Donahue appears to support their points of view, and his producers have turned down rebuttal requests from the scientific community.

Many people who have heard of the "fairness doctrine" wonder whether the Federal Communications Commission (FCC) could help the scientific community counteract the excessive amount of nutrition misinformation which is broadcast on these programs. Although FCC policies are designed to promote open discussion of public controversies, the agency also wished to avoid "censorship." The FCC will intervene when needed to assure exposure of opposing viewpoints in *political* campaigns. But it will not intervene in controversies over "truth in news" unless there is clearcut evidence of "intentional falsification" by a broadcaster. Nor is the FCC usually concerned with the content of major talk shows—which it regards as "entertainment."

Most local TV and radio talk shows give unbalanced coverage to health food industry promoters—not because they are biased, but

for a different reason. There are many more promoters than opponents suggesting themselves as guests! The typical talk show
guest is someone who has written a popular book, who is being
promoted by a professional public relations firm, and who can
spend considerable amounts of time publicizing his ideas because
book sales will repay him for the time. Health food industry
opponents are rarely in this position. Some opponents are willing
to appear on talk shows in their home communities and in other
cities when they attend professional meetings. But virtually all of
them have other professional duties (teaching, research or patient
care) which limit their availability for public appearances.

The Threat of Libel

Another factor which dampens professional enthusiasm for
fighting misinformation is the fear of being sued. Libel suits can be
costly to defend, and some health food promoters are inclined to
be litigious.

In 1959, Fredrick J. Stare, M.D., professor of nutrition at Harvard
University, was sued for libel by the Boston Nutrition Society. The
issue arose after Dr. Stare commented in *McCall's* magazine on
claims by the Society that white bread was devoid of nutrients and
was related to the development of heart disease and cancer. He
characterized such claims as "a cruel and reckless fraud."

The case eventually came to trial before a jury which deliberated
only 15 minutes before ruling in Stare's favor. The trial judge
instructed the jury that "A professional person ... has a privilege in
his field of competence to differ with others supposedly in the
same field, to speak out strongly, as long as his comments are not
made with malice."

In 1973, several leaders of the National Nutritional Foods Association (NNFA) sued the FDA and the Department of Health, Education and Welfare for $500 million, claiming that adverse
publicity from these agencies had damaged their businesses. The
district court ruled that "defamation" of an entire industry is not
grounds for suit and dismissed the complaint. One of the plaintiffs
in this suit was Sid Cammy, owner of a health food store in New
Jersey called The Diet Shop. In February 1978, he included the
following comments in a column in *Health Foods Business*:

> If you recall, last month I spoke about taking deadly mea-
> sures with telling effect. And so I shall.
> ... Use every means at your disposal. Find out how our side
> can get before the public eye on every front, to inflict hard-

hitting lightning blows against the attackers. Should they say a product is dangerous, we will say it is one of the safest foods in the world and that 90% of the foods sold in supermarkets should have warning labels . . .

The so-called experts who knock health foods are paid hirelings or have close ties with the food and drug industries. The fact that these people have impressive degrees should not blind anyone to the fact that scientific quackery is still quackery . . .

Let our Industry challenge these folks to prove what they say and then let them have it with both barrels. Expose the agencies! Expose the personnel! . . . Demand a Congressional investigation regarding their connections and activities. They must be put on the defensive.

We must never go into any battle as shoeshine boys or inferiors . . . With these plans in mind, we have a fair chance to rout our enemies when the final assault comes. And it is coming.

Several months later, NNFA launched "Operation Counterattack," a new strategy against critics of the health food industry. "Phase One" was a suit against Sheriff John F. Duffy of San Diego County, charging that a booklet he was distributing contained false criticisms of the health food industry. The case did not come to trial because the booklet, *Beware Health "Quackery"*, was discontinued by its publisher.

NNFA's next step was a suit against Dr. Stare and his associate, Elizabeth M. Whelan, Sc.D., executive director of the American Council on Science and Health. The suit, filed jointly by NNFA, Cammy and two other NNFA officers who owned health food stores, charged the two scientists with conspiring to "defame, injure, disparage, damage and destroy the reputation and business of plaintiffs." Through books and published articles, the suit claimed, Drs. Stare and Whelan had "recklessly, maliciously and knowingly disseminated false and defamatory remarks with respect to plaintiffs and the health food industry."

Nutrition scientists all over America responded to this suit with outrage. It was obvious that plaintiffs could not win the suit in court. Their names hadn't even been mentioned in the publications to which they were objecting. Seeing the suit as a threat to the freedom of expression of all nutrition scientists, nutrition organizations and friends of the defendants raised enough money to pay for the suit's defense.

To prove libel under the laws of New York State (where the Stare-Whelan suit was filed), it is necessary to show that a defendant used defamatory words against plaintiffs that were untrue and that caused measurable damages. Federal Judge Abraham D. Sofaer, who dismissed the case in 1980, ruled that plaintiffs had met none of these requirements. He also warned that "any further suit by plaintiffs against critics of the health food industry should be scrutinized carefully to determine whether it was brought in good faith."

Do you think NNFA officials believed they could win any of their libel suits in court? Or do you think their purpose was to discourage criticism of the health food industry? More important, how much should nutrition scientists be intimidated by the threat of libel?

We believe that scientists who understand the law and use common sense have little to fear. One cannot libel an *idea*. Therefore it is not libelous to attack an idea or to list the charactistic signs of quackery or to say that something is "questionable." One cannot libel a large group of individuals or an entire industry. One can libel an *individual* (or an organization) by engaging in name-calling. Therefore you should never call anyone a name (like "quack") unless you are willing to defend this claim in court. It is legal to mention relevant adverse *facts* about someone who places himself in the public spotlight by claiming to have expert knowledge. But avoid statements about *motivation* (such as "He's only in it for the money") because they may be impossible to prove.

Is it likely that anyone who follows these rules will be sued? In our opinion it is not. Very few libel suits have actually been filed by health food industry proponents because the likelihood of winning in court is virtually zero. If an industry-wide policy of suing critics just to harass them should arise, two things are likely to happen. First the scientific community will rally to help those being sued. Then the courts will begin to order unsuccessful plaintiffs to pay the costs of defense.

Peer Review?

In Chapter 1 of this book, we describe how scientists are eager to point out the deficiencies in each other's theories and experimental techniques. This process of "peer review" is basic to scientific growth and the establishment of "scientific truth." The comparable "goal" of journalism is to report what happens. *Journalists almost never publicly criticize each other's coverage of the news.* This is particularly true when health topics are involved.

Have you ever seen a letter to the editor from a reporter who charged that his own newspaper or magazine misled the public in an article or advertisement about health? Have you ever heard a radio or TV commentator state that misinformation about health was broadcast on his station? Have you ever seen an editorial in print which charged that a health topic was mishandled by another publication?

Recently, when the journalistic community discovered that a Pulitzer Prize-winning story was a fake, there were many editorial expressions of outrage. Have you ever seen an expression of editorial outrage directed against poor reporting which might cause thousands of unsuspecting people to become victims of quackery? Carol Burnett's libel suit against the *National Enquirer* was one of the biggest news events of 1981. Has any newspaper or magazine ever warned its readers that the "miracle" nutrition claims found frequently in the *Enquirer* and similar publications may not be worth the paper they are printed on? As far as we know, except for *Consumer Reports*, the answer is no.

The National News Council

There is one journalistic peer review agency which can sometimes help to counteract misinformation in the news media: The National News Council, One Lincoln Plaza, New York, NY 10023. Founded in 1973, the Council has as its purpose "to serve the public interest by . . . advancing accurate and fair reporting of news." Toward this end, it investigates complaints alleging unfairness, inaccuracy or breaches of ethical standards by wire services, newspapers, news syndicates, news magazines and television and radio networks and stations. It does not (unfortunately) involve itself with the fairness of talk shows.

The Council confines its examinations of such complaints to national news media, except when it believes that local coverage is of national significance. It concerns itself with editorial comment only when allegations of fact are in dispute. Most of the thousands of complaints received so far have been informally resolved. Major cases are reported in *Columbia Journalism Review*, a magazine which is widely read by writers and editors. Here are some examples:

In 1976, Dr. Stephen Barrett complained about a column attacking fluoridation, written by Ralph DeToledano and distributed by Copley News Service. When Copley learned of the complaint, it invited Dr. Barrett to submit an article about fluoridation's benefits for distribution to 800 newspapers. The syndicate's editor, who agreed that DeToledano's column was inaccurate, also promised Dr. Barrett that no similar column would be distributed in the future. Satisfied that "fairness" had been achieved, the National News Council decided not to involve itself in judging the accuracy of DeToledano's original article.

In 1977, Dr. Barrett complained about an article in *Parade* magazine suggesting that Dr. J. Anthony Morris had been fired from the FDA because he opposed the swine flu program. This matter is significant because the Morris case is being misrepresented as evidence that the FDA should not be trusted in health matters. Morris was actually dismissed for "insubordination" and "inefficiency" by an administrative process begun more than six months before he spoke out against the flu program. Ruling that "an essential element of the story was clearly missing," the National News Council upheld Dr. Barrett's complaint. A few months later, when the *New York Times Magazine* carried a similarly one-sided account of Morris's firing, Dr. Barrett again complained to the Council and was upheld. In 1981, *Parade* carried another article claiming that Morris was dismissed for "blowing the whistle." Dr. Barrett complained again, but the Council has not yet ruled.

In 1978, Eleanor M. Fala, a registered dietitian from Havertown, Pennsylvania, complained that the *Philadelphia Bulletin* was acting in a biased manner by giving favorable coverage to many questionable "nutrition" theories while ignoring protests from the local scientific community. Although the Council did not uphold the complaint, the newspaper did respond by publishing more articles which were scientifically accurate.

In 1980, Dr. Victor Herbert joined Dr. Barrett in complaining that an article in *Us* magazine gave unwarranted respectability to Kurt Donsbach and his mail-order nutrition school. "It's the real thing," the writer had claimed, "the first—and so far only—university in the country dealing with the various aspects of nutrition." The Council upheld the complaint, concluding that "*Us* magazine made Dr. Donsbach and his university appear to meet conventional standards that even Dr. Donsbach does not claim for himself or his school."

In 1981, Dr. Herbert charged that an article in *People* magazine misled the public by giving the appearance of reliability for Richard Passwater and his "doctoral" degree from Bernadean University (see Chapter 4). Herbert charged further that despite his warnings to one of its authors, the article falsely suggested that large quantities of vitamins, selenium and zinc are safe and beneficial. After determining that Bernadean University had no authority to grant degrees in the states where it operated, the Council concluded that *People* had "failed to exercise elementary and necessary journalistic responsibility that would have put the public on notice." It should have checked Passwater's academic credentials and included its findings in the article.

What Else Can be Done?

Professionals who have expert knowledge of nutrition can influence their local media by letting reporters, editors and producers know that they are available for consultation. If inaccurate information is published or broadcast, a well-reasoned letter or phone call to a reporter, editor or station manager may lead to publication of accurate information. It is important to realize, however, that many media executives are influenced more by the number of people who care than by the logic of the arguments presented. A coordinated effort by many concerned citizens will often have far more effect than the actions of one individual.

Many people would like to see something done but are afraid to become involved in public controversy. These people can still help by indicating their concerns by telephone or by writing letters marked "not for publication."

Professional groups can sponsor community-wide educational programs. Two of the most popular are Dial-A-Dietitian telephone consultation services and medical TV talk shows organized by county medical societies. Speakers' bureaus should also be organized. To be most effective, professionals who communicate to the public should undergo formal training in public speaking.

Health scientists must learn to speak out more against nutrition misinformation that is rampant in the media. Somehow we must find a way to arouse public indignation against the vitamin peddlers who have been hustling them. It would help a great deal if we could persuade media executives to care more about how their actions can affect people's health.

Chapter 12

The Weakness of the Law

Don't make the mistake of thinking that the law forces people to tell the truth about nutrition products. It is perfectly legal to tell a lie in a publication or on a talk show as long as you are not selling the product at the same time. It is not legal to make false claims on the label of a product, in an advertisement, or during a direct sale; but as we shall see, prosecution of law violators is quite limited.

Three federal agencies—the Postal Service, the FDA and the FTC—can act against false claims made by sellers of food supplements.

Postal Laws

The Postal Service has jurisdiction over situations where the mail is used to transfer money for products or services. Postal inspectors look for misleading advertisements in magazines and newspapers and on radio or television. They also receive complaints from the public and from other government agencies.

Title 39, Section 3005, of the United States Code can be used to block promoters of misleading schemes from receiving money through the mail. If sufficient health hazard or economic detriment exists, an immediate court order to impound mail may be sought under Section 3007 of the Code. Title 18, Section 1341, provides for criminal prosecution. The maximum penalties are a fine of $1,000, five years in prison, or both, for each instance proved. Under this section, intent to deceive must be proved—a task which can be difficult and time-consuming. Though Section 1341 is used sparingly in medical cases, almost all cases actually brought to trial result in convictions.

Criminal cases, consent agreements and false representation orders (which stop mail delivery) are noted in the *Law Enforcement Report* which is issued three times a year, free-of-charge, to interested media and consumer protection agencies.

FDA Laws

The U.S. Food and Drug Administration (FDA) traces its roots to just after the turn of this century, when consumers needed all the protection they could get. Patent medicines, which were worthless but not always harmless, were widely promoted with cure-all claims. The country was plagued by unsanitary conditions in meat-packing plants. Harmful chemicals were being added to foods, and labels rarely told what their products contained.

The Pure Food and Drug Act, passed in 1906, has been strengthened by a number of amendments and related acts. Together, these various laws are concerned with assuring the safety and effectiveness of all products intended for use in the diagnosis, prevention and treatment of disease. The 1938 Food, Drug and Cosmetic Act bans false and misleading statements from the labeling of foods, drugs and medical devices. Drugs must have their active ingredients listed and be proven safe before marketing. The Kefauver-Harris Drug Amendments (passed in 1962 in the wake of the Thalidomide tragedy) require that drugs must also be proven *effective* before marketing. The Medical Device Amendments of 1976 extend this requirement to many devices.

Under the law, "labeling" is not limited to what is on a product's container. It also includes claims made by any written or graphic matter which explains a product's use and is physically or contextually connected with its sale. Thus promotional material used to sell a product or to explain its use can be labeling whether it is used before or after a sale.

The FDA's jurisdiction covers all of a product's intended uses whether they are contained in labeling or not. Section 502(f)(1) of the Food, Drug and Cosmetic Act requires that all drugs and devices bear adequate directions for use. Someone who attempts to build a market for a quack remedy through oral claims or promotion through the media can be stopped by use of Section 501(f)(1) plus Regulation 201.128 which requires labeling to contain adequate directions for all *intended* uses whether promotion is done by oral claims, advertising or otherwise.

Complaints about quack remedies are usually received from consumers, members of Congress, FDA field inspectors and various government agencies. Significant complaints may be followed up by FDA field inspectors and evaluated by physicians and other scientists. If investigation shows that a product is a "new drug," it must have FDA approval for movement in interstate commerce. Violation of this provision can lead to seizure of the product and a court injunction against its sale.

To be classified as a "new drug," a product does not actually have to be new. It can also be a familiar substance proposed for a therapeutic use that is "not generally recognized as safe and effective." For example, a claim that wheat germ oil "prevents heart stress" would make the oil a new drug with respect to that claim. The oil would also be misbranded because the seller could not provide adequate directions to achieve the intended effect.

It is a criminal offense to market a drug that is unapproved or misbranded. A first offender may be fined up to $1,000, imprisoned up to one year, or both. Any offense committed after a first conviction is a felony punishable by a fine up to $10,000 and three years in prison. Because misbranding and marketing an unapproved new drug are separate offenses, a repeat offender could be penalized by a fine of up to $20,000 and six years in jail. To obtain a conviction, intent to mislead need not be proved. Even a single shipment of a single product is sufficient grounds for conviction. Before criminal action is begun, however, offenders are often given a chance to withdraw their product from the market or to change its labeling; and in cases of minor violations, civil action is usually taken.

The *FDA Consumer*, which is available by subscription, describes many of the FDA's consumer protection activities. It is an excellent magazine with good articles each month about food safety and "nutrition" ripoffs.

FTC Laws

The Federal Trade Commission (FTC) was established in 1914. Its original purpose was to safeguard businesses against monopoly and unfair competition. Five Commissioners who serve staggered terms head this agency. Control of health quackery was not a major concern of the early Commissioners. With the appointment of William E. Humphrey in 1925, there was a marked increase in the attack on false drug advertising. But until passage of the Wheeler-Lea Act in 1938, agency emphasis was on injury to competitors rather than consumers.

The FTC has jurisdiction over advertising of foods, non-prescription drugs, cosmetics and devices that are sold or advertised in interstate commerce. Section 12 of the Wheeler-Lea Act allows the government to attack false advertising which could injure consumers as well as competitors. In determining what is false, what is left out may be considered as well as what is said. If a problem is serious enough, a court injunction can halt the practice being challenged until the matter can be resolved under regular administrative procedure.

The FTC has broad powers to investigate complaints. Uncooperative businessmen—who do not answer questions, reveal documents or respond to subpoena—are subject to heavy penalties. If investigation concludes that a law violation exists, the FTC may issue a Complaint. At this point, advertisers may comply voluntarily without admitting wrongdoing. If they resist, an Administrative Law Judge will hold a hearing which can lead to a "cease-and-desist" order. Such orders become final if not appealed to the Commission. Commission decisions, in turn, are subject to appeal through federal courts.

Cease-and-desist orders set forth findings and prohibit respondents from engaging in practices determined to be illegal. When final, these orders act as permanent injunctions. Penalties for violating consent agreements or cease-and-desist orders can be very heavy—including prison sentences, corrective advertising, and fines up to $10,000 per day for continued violations. In 1976, for example, the J. B. Williams Company paid $302,000 as a result of violating cease-and-desist orders which prohibit various false claims for *Geritol* and *FemIron*, two of its patent medicines.

In addition to cease-and-desist orders, the FTC issues industry guides and trade regulation rules. Guides are interpretive statements without the force of law. Rules represent the conclusions of the Commission about what it considers unlawful. Once a rule is established, lengthy explanations of the reasons why a particular ad is unfair or deceptive are no longer necessary. A reference to the rule is enough. Before guides and rules are established, interested parties are given the opportunity to comment.

A 1980 amendment of the FTC Act requires the agency to publish every six months a 12-month forecast of rules it intends to propose or adopt. Before any rule can go into effect, however, it must also be presented to Congress for 90 days—where a veto by either house will kill it. Called the "FTC Improvements Act," this law is the result of intense lobbying by the funeral industry and other special interest groups who wished to weaken FTC action against their deceptive practices.

Three trade regulation rules that involve the health food industry have been under consideration during the past six years. Guidelines have been proposed for testimonial advertising, protein supplements and food advertising (including "health," "organic" and "natural" food claims). Unfortunately, it appears that the proposed standards for "natural" claims will increase deception of consumers rather than prevent it (see Chapter 7).

The FTC's activities are reported in the weekly *FTC News Summary* and an annual report which are available free-of-charge to interested parties.

Effectiveness

Most people believe that claims for health products must be true or else "they wouldn't be allowed." We wish that were so. The laws described above are potentially very powerful, but it is important to understand their limitations.

Enforcement of postal laws is sufficiently effective that in recent years, few mail-order companies have been making direct false claims that nutrients can prevent or treat various conditions. Similarly, FDA enforcement of "new drug" laws had discouraged the use of false health claims *directly* on product labels. But the health food industry has very little need to make its claims in direct advertising or on actual labels. News articles, books, magazine articles and radio and TV talk shows have done such a good sales job that most people "*know*" what food supplements are supposed to be good for. False and misleading oral claims are also being made in the privacy of health food stores, the homes of customers, the offices of questionable practitioners, and sometimes even at accredited educational meetings for health professionals.

About 10 years ago, the Lehigh Valley Committee Against Health Fraud asked a local FDA agent whether he would like committee members to gather tape-recorded evidence for prosecution of local health food store owners who had been observed making false claims to their customers. The agent replied that the FDA prefers to use its limited resources to regulate labeling claims by manufacturers and major distributors. Prosecution of "little" storekeepers by "big" government would be both impractical and politically unpopular.

Actually, the FDA appears to ignore most cases of food supplement misbranding which are brought to its attention. During the past 10 years, the Lehigh Valley Committee Against Health Fraud has brought more than 100 misbranded products to the attention of the FDA. Not one prosecution took place as a result. Even when a committee member actually made a "buy" at the request of an FDA official as a preliminary step to criminal prosecution of a distributor, prosecution did not take place! According to FDA officials, agency priority is being given to assuring the safety and effectiveness of legitimate drugs. Only the most notorious quack remedies—such as laetrile, "B_{15}" and Gerovital GH3—have been the object of visible enforcement activity.

The FTC appears to be even less interested in food supplement advertising. Ads which suggest that a daily vitamin or vitamin-mineral supplement be taken "to be sure" or for "nutritional insurance" are apparently not misleading enough to inspire corrective action by the FTC. Nor are the ads for *Stresstabs* and similar products which suggest falsely that people under "stress" need nutrients beyond those obtainable from a balanced diet. Despite repeated complaints, the FTC has also resisted going after the fake "vitamin," B_{15}.

Newspapers and general circulation magazines occasionally carry ads for nutrient products falsely claimed to retard aging or improve hair, nails or skin. The largest promoter of such products appears to be Cosvetic Laboratories, a subsidiary of Braswell, Inc., of Atlanta, Georgia. Other company names used by this organization include Quest Research, Peak Labs, Head Start, Standard Research Labs and Earthquest Ltd. *Body Forum*, a magazine published by A. Glenn Braswell, describes itself as "an owner's manual for your body . . . America's most prominent health care magazine." Promising to provide its readers with "the best and most incredible preventive health information," the magazine contains articles and advertisements which make miraculous claims for a wide variety of "natural" products.

A 1-year subscription to *Body Forum* costs $10, but buyers of $9.50 or more from Cosvetic Laboratories get a free 18-month subscription. During 1980, the magazine carried ads for about 50 different products, such as: *RNA Cream* ("to fight wrinkles"), *Formula 40* ("to restore hair"), *BEZ-P39* (a supposed breast enlargement plan "which teams digestive aids with special enzymes," a protein formula and exercises), *Vitagland*, (glandular extracts with "remarkable youth-sustaining properties"), *Bio-Genesis* ("for germinating new hair growth on previously bald heads"), *The Man's Vitamin* ("to make sure you get the nutrients essential to healthy sexual functioning"), *Superoxide Dismutase* ("if you'd rather not grow old before your time"), *Nature's Sleeping Pill*, ("absolutely non-habit forming"), *Neocel* ("to improve cell quality"), *Bio-NC 36* ("to bring hair follicles back to life") and *Formula 12 Creme* ("to get rid of stubborn cellulite").

Braswell's products can be ordered by mail or charged to a credit card by calling a toll-free number. They are also being sold on a person-to-person basis and in health food stores and pharmacies.

In 1980, the Postal Service took action against more than 20 products sold by the $20 million-a-year Braswell conglomerate, including most of the products listed above. Orders sent through the mail for many of these products were stopped and returned to their senders, but telephone orders are outside of Postal Service jurisdiction. The Atlanta office of the FDA also took action. In response to its warnings, Braswell's attorney promised "tighter editorial control" over *Body Forum* and an end to certain product claims. Current issues of the magazine contain an almost entirely new product line, but claims for these products are still false or misleading. The company has transferred some of its operations from Georgia to Florida, but the Postal Service remains in hot pursuit. Recently the FTC filed a complaint charging that ads for three Braswell products were misleading, and that the company failed to issue refunds under money-back guarantees advertised in *Cosmopolitan, Penthouse, Psychology Today, Us, Vogue, Star, The National Enquirer,* and *Women's Wear Daily.* But money will continue to roll in while these cases proceed slowly through the courts.

A few companies that make questionable claims for products like enzymes, chelated minerals, "glandulars" and homeopathic remedies market them primarily through chiropractors. Contact with the chiropractors is made through direct mailings, company-sponsored seminars and advertisements in chiropractic journals. The FDA, which could easily prosecute manufacturers or distributors of these products for misbranding, has shown no recent interest in this area. In 1976, successful criminal action was taken against Linblads, Inc., a distributor located in Dearborn, Michigan; but as far as we know, *this is the only such criminal prosecution in more than 15 years!*

In 1975, the Lehigh Valley Committee Against Health Fraud complained to the Postal Service about Metabolic Products, a California firm operated by Kurt Donsbach (see Chapter 10). Although the company appeared to be using the mails to sell misbranded products to chiropractors, the postal authorities declined to intervene. Recently we asked attorney George C. Davis of the Postal Service's Consumer Protection Division why no prosecution had taken place. He replied:

> Unfortunately our files no longer contain any information on this case. Based, however, on the Inspection Service memorandum which you supplied, I would think it likely that we concluded that few of the recipients of this advertising (chiropractors) would be misled by the promoter's claims and that our efforts might be more beneficially expended elsewhere.

We do not adhere to the view that "there is no such thing as false advertising to licensed health professionals because they are supposedly capable of distinguishing fact from fiction." Looking over the material you furnished, it would seem likely that we concluded that in view of the relative sophistication of the recipients of this advertising and the relative absurdity of many of its claims, there was less likelihood of significant public injury than was apparent in other schemes then pending before us. With our limited resources, we simply cannot act against all advertising schemes which appear to violate 39 U.S.C. 3005; and when we are in the position—as we usually are—of having more potential cases than we can handle, we try to pick and choose among the cases based upon our best guess as to the potential harm the scheme might cause.

A product seizure or criminal prosecution by the FDA is likely to have far more effect than a series of mail-stop actions by the Postal Service. But as noted above, *the FDA gives very little priority to protecting Americans from misbranded food supplements.*

State Regulation

Healing arts practitioners who resell products in their offices are usually subject to state rather than federal jurisdiction. Unfortunately, if a practitioner is licensed, state agencies usually have little interest in what treatment he recommends unless he kills a patient. The lack of interest applies not only to chiropractors and naturopaths, but also to the small number of medical doctors, dentists and others who use bizarre types of questionable remedies. Practitioners who prescribe huge doses of vitamins, or who use hair analysis, muscle testing or computer analysis of diet as a basis for recommending food supplements, encounter little or no interference from state governments.

Federal agencies also lack jurisdiction over the sale of questionable remedies that are manufactured and sold entirely within the borders of a state. Most states have laws which could be used to stop the sale of such drugs, but enforcement of these laws is generally given low priority. A few state legislatures—most notably Nevada's—appear to regard the availability of questionable remedies as a tourist attraction!

As noted in Chapter 4, most health food stores are willing to offer advice to their customers. Although "diagnosis" and "treatment" are illegal, agencies in most states ignore the sales tactics used in these stores. Perhaps if more people who realize they have been victimized were to complain about it, law enforcement authorities would take the situation more seriously. In California, which may be the only state that uses undercover investigators, a few storekeepers have been prosecuted for practicing medicine without a license; but in 1978, the health food industry gained passage of a law allowing anyone to give "nutritional advice" as long as it does not constitute diagnosis or treatment.

Civil Remedies

Nutrition authorities have documented cases where excess vitamins or minerals have harmed people. How many preachers of nutrition gospel have ever mentioned this fact on a radio or television talk show? This deception by omission should be prosecuted as negligence chargeable not only to the huckster, but also to his talk show host and sponsoring network. It seems possible that "reckless endangerment" laws could be revised or interpreted to include endangerment of public health by promotion of dangerous nutritional practices. We also wonder whether the more dangerous of the quack's misrepresentations could be enjoined as a public nuisance. Perhaps a public-spirited prosecutor will try these approaches someday. If the First Amendment does not protect smut speech and writings which are alleged to injure mental health, why should it protect misleading "nutrition" claims that can be *proven* harmful to physical health? It is not legal to shout "Fire!" in a crowded theater where no fire exists. Do you think that other misinformation which can kill people deserves protection under our First Amendment?

Under our civil laws, it should be possible for a private citizen to recover substantial damages if he is harmed by reliance upon misinformation purveyed by a self-appointed "nutrition expert." The citizen would need to establish that the "expert" has a duty not to mislead him. If a licensed physician recommends a remedy, he has a duty to use care in selecting it and to warn of complications. If a patient is harmed because his doctor fails to do either of these things, he can sue for malpractice. Is it too much to expect that an unlicensed promoter of quackery can be held responsible for the harm he does?

A California case has created a precedent that can be cited by anyone who has been harmed by following the advice of a nutrition quack when given in a broadcast. In *Weirum vs. RKO General, Inc.*, the Supreme Court of California upheld a jury verdict of $300,000 against a radio station. The station had offered a cash prize to the first person who could locate a traveling disc jockey. Two teenagers spotted the disc jockey and tried to follow him to a contest stopping point. During the pursuit, one of the cars was forced off the road, killing its driver. The jury found that the broadcast had *created a foreseeable risk* to motorists because its contest conditions could stimulate accidents. Many radio and television stations which broadcast nutrition quackery have been put on notice by scientists that they are creating an unreasonable risk of harm. Such stations might have serious difficulty defending themselves against suits by injured listeners.

In 1976, the estate of Adelle Davis paid $150,000 to settle out-of-court a suit brought by Mrs. Katherine Young of Maine on behalf of her daughter, Eliza. The child had been given "generous amounts of vitamin A" during her first year of life as recommended in Ms. Davis' book *Let's Have Healthy Children*. The result was a permanent stunting of her growth. Another suit was filed in Florida in 1979 against the book's publisher by the parents of Ryan Pitzer. According to the suit, Ryan was killed at two months of age by the administration of "health food" potassium chloride for colic as suggested in the book. Since the *majority* of "nutrition" books sold to the public contain misinformation which is potentially dangerous, the outcome of this lawsuit may be of monumental significance to the publishing industry.

What Else Is Needed?

It is clear that promoters of nutrition misinformation have a very broad base of operations which cannot be completely contained no matter how vigorously or imaginatively our laws are written or enforced. But some aspects of the vitamin and health food hustle could be crippled by appropriate government action.

Consumers Union has suggested passage of a law giving the Postal Service the power to assess civil penalties equal to or greater than the profits of mail-order thieves. Such a measure would eliminate the financial incentive to individual promoters. It would also be a good idea to give the Postal Service the power to assess similar penalties against the publishers of misleading ads. This could eliminate the financial incentive to publish such ads.

Many publishers claim that ad screening is too cumbersome, but there is no truth to such assertion. Many publications already do an effective job of it. Any publisher who wishes to do so can easily locate a trustworthy nutrition scientist who would screen prospective ads rapidly and free-of-charge. The Lehigh Valley Committee Against Health Fraud has offered such service to many publishers, but so far has had no takers. Publishers could also develop industry standards and set up a clearinghouse to keep track of common false claims and companies that have already violated the law. Such information is easily obtainable.

If the publishing industry does not establish self-regulation, the FTC could develop a trade regulation rule to force publishers to adopt responsible screening standards. Laws could also be passed so that publishers of false ads can share in any civil or criminal liability of the advertiser. If medical doctors who have years of training are legally accountable for their medical advice, and if hospitals are sometimes held accountable for the negligence of their staff, why should publishers be able to disseminate unsafe medical advice with no liability whatsoever? Vigorous FTC action is also needed against food supplement manufacturers who use subtle but misleading scare tactics in magazine ads and on television.

Another good approach is now being tried by the government of Belgium. In 1980, the Belgian Parliament passed a law to stop certain advertisers from claiming that their products have medical properties or effects. Food advertisers will no longer be permitted to use such words as "natural," "pure," "low-calorie," "medical" or "organic." The new law forbids the representation on food labels of body organs or the use of imagery which falsely suggests endorsement by the medical, dental, pharmaceutical or nursing professions. It will also be unlawful to induce consumers to believe that a product or brand possesses particular qualities when, in fact, all similar food products have the same qualities.

Questionable remedies marketed through licensed practitioners or media promotions could be virtually driven off the market by vigorous enforcement of labeling laws by the FDA. More than anything else, *criminal* prosecution by the FDA—with *imprisonment* of major lawbreakers—is urgently needed to stem the rising tide of nutritional quackery in America.

Quite frankly, we are not optimistic that any of the above consumer protection measures will be carried out in the United States in the foreseeable future. In fact an opposite trend is apparent. Although quackery is increasing, too many government officials do not see it as a serious problem which deserves priority. *Caveat emptor* ("Let the buyer beware") is again becoming the law of the land.

Ultimately, your best protection will be your own good sense. If the majority of American physicians wouldn't use a product or give it to their loved ones, you shouldn't use it either.

Chapter 13

Where to Get Help

In most professions, educational standards are controlled by licensing laws which protect the public. But in nutrition, anyone who so chooses can declare himself an "expert." We have already discussed the training (or lack of it) of phonies. This chapter tells how real experts are trained and how you can get reliable advice.

If you have a question about nutrition, the most convenient person to ask is probably your own physician. Doctors are often accused of not knowing much about nutrition. This charge usually comes from food faddists who would like everyone to believe that they are the experts while physicians are nutritional illiterates. It also comes from patients who are disappointed when their doctors correctly inform them that "supernutrition" is not the key to "superhealth" and that "some is good" does not mean "more is better." Nutrition, after all, is *part* of medicine, not a *substitute* for it.

The principles of nutrition are those of human biochemistry and physiology, courses required in every medical school. There are substantial sections on nutrition in every standard textbook of medicine, surgery, obstetrics and pediatrics used in the United States. Most medical schools do not teach a separate required course in nutrition, but this does not mean the subject is ignored. Most medical educators prefer that nutrition be taught in other courses, at the points where it is most relevant. For example, nutrition in growth and development is taught in pediatrics, nutrition in wound healing is taught in surgery, and nutrition in pregnancy is covered in obstetrics. In addition, 70 percent of the schools now offer an elective course in nutrition. Fundamental to the training of all physicians is the axiom that no product should be considered safe and effective until *proved* to be safe and effective.

A physician's training, of course, does not end on the day of graduation from medical school or completion of specialty training. The medical profession advocates *lifelong* education, and physicians can further their knowledge of nutrition by reading medical journals, discussing cases with colleagues and attending continuing education courses. Virtually all physicians know what nutrients can and cannot do and can tell the difference between a real nutritional discovery and a piece of quack nonsense. If your doctor is unable to answer your question, he can refer you to someone who will—often a registered dietitian.

Respectable Credentials

Nutrition courses offered at accredited universities are based on scientific principles and taught by qualified instructors. A bachelor's degree requires four years of full-time study which qualify a graduate for entry level positions in dietetics or food service, often in a hospital. A masters degree in nutrition, which can widen career opportunities and improve chances for advancement, requires two more years of full-time study beyond the undergraduate level.

People who wish to become nutrition researchers usually pursue a Ph.D. in biochemistry. This requires a minimum of two years of additional study plus a thesis based on original laboratory research. Those wishing to concentrate on teaching or educational research usually seek the degrees of Ph.D. or Ed.D. in nutrition education. A nutrition education dissertation will be less oriented toward laboratory research than one in science, but must still provide an original contribution to the field of nutrition education.

Each nutrition-related degree earned from an accredited university signifies that a person has a broad background in science of nutrition and a thorough grasp of nutritional concepts.

In addition to an academic degree, most legitimate nutritionists seek professional certification. There are two professional associations which are restricted to qualified nutrition scientists. Active membership in the American Institute of Nutrition (AIN) is open to respected scientists who have published meritorious original research on some aspect of nutrition, who are presently working in the field, and who are sponsored by two AIN members. Nominees are considered by a membership committee, a council of officers, and the membership. The clinical arm of AIN is the American Society for Clinical Nutrition (ASCN), which has similar requirements but specifies clinical research. All ASCN members are also members of AIN, and about 70 percent of them are physicians. Promoters of nutrition quackery are not admitted to membership in AIN or ASCN.

Nutritionists at the doctoral level may also seek certification by the American Board of Nutrition as specialists in clinical nutrition

(M.D.s only) or human nutritional sciences (M.D.s and Ph.D.s). There are currently about 400 board-certified nutrition specialists in the U.S., all of whom have passed an examination on all aspects of nutrition including deficiency diseases, toxicity of excess vitamins, metabolism, food-drug interactions, therapeutic diets, and the significance of the Recommended Dietary Allowances. Promoters of nutrition quackery are not qualified to take this examination. Certified nutritionists usually work in medical schools and hospitals, where they conduct clinical research and offer consultation to primary care physicians.

Registered dietitians (R.D.s) are specially trained to translate nutrition research into healthful, tasty diets. Compared to physicians, they usually know less about basic biochemistry, physiology and metabolism, but more about the nutrient content of specific foods. The R.D. certification is usually sought by bachelor and master level nutrition graduates. To qualify, they must have additional professional experience and pass a comprehensive written test covering all aspects of nutrition and food service management. They must also participate regularly in continuing education programs approved by the American Dietetic Association.

Most of the country's 35,000 active R.D.s work in hospitals. Typically, they counsel patients and conduct classes for pregnant women, heart and kidney patients, diabetics, and other persons with special dietary needs. Dietitians are also employed by community agencies such as geriatric, day care, and drug/alcohol abuse centers. Some dietitians do research. Others engage in private practice where they counsel physician-referred clients.

How to Write for Help

A number of organizations evaluate and publish accurate information about nutrition. Some serve and communicate primarily with health and nutrition professionals, while others communicate primarily with the public. Should you write to any of them for information, keep in mind that the individual who receives your letter is likely to be extremely busy. You will be most likely to get a helpful response if you do the following:

1. Type your letter to assure legibility.
2. Ask your question in as brief but specific a way as possible.
3. Tell something about yourself and why you need the information. Briefly indicate what you already know or have read.
4. Enclose a large enough stamped, self-addressed envelope.

Government Agencies

• The Food and Drug Administration will answer inquiries and has available a variety of educational materials about nutrition and nutritional quackery. Its consumer affairs offices, located in 30 major cities, can furnish speakers for interested groups. The FDA is also interested in receiving complaints about food supplement products which are sold with false claims or inadequate directions for use. Its address is 5600 Fishers Lane, Rockville, MD 20857.

• The Postal Service can act against products sold through the mails with false claims. Complaints should be sent to the Fraud Division, Chief U.S. Postal Inspector, Washington, DC 20260.

• The Federal Trade Commission has jurisdiction over advertising which is false or misleading. Complaints should be addressed to the FTC Bureau of Consumer Protection, Washington, DC 20580.

• The U.S. Department of Agriculture, which developed the concept of basic food groups so important in teaching of sound nutrition, can answer questions and provide literature on nutrition and diet. Write: Food and Nutrition Information Center, USDA National Agricultural Library, Room 304, 10301 Baltimore Blvd., Beltsville, MD 20705, or telephone 301-344-3719 between 8:00AM and 4:30PM, EST.

• The USDA Extension Service of each land-grant university can answer questions about nutrition. Home economists at USDA county cooperative services can answer questions about food preparation. Your local telephone directory can tell you if your community has either of these two services available.

• The Department of Health and Human Services (HHS, formerly HEW) has several nutrition services. Its Administration on Children, Youth and Families (ACYF) administers the Head Start Program and develops nutrition education materials and services for parents of low-income families. The ACYF central office is located at Donohoe Building, 400 6th St., S.W., Washington, DC 20024. Contact with local Head Start programs can be made through your local school system. HHS's Administration on Aging provides services to persons 60 years of age or older. Both national and regional offices provide publications and other information. They also make referrals to state and local offices which provide group meals, home delivered meals and nutrition education. The national office is located at 330 Independence Ave., S.W., Washington, DC 20201. In addition a broad range of nutrition publications and information is available from the Health Services Administration of the U.S. Public Health Service, Washington, DC 20852, and U.S. Government Printing Office, Pueblo, CO 81009.

• The National Institute for Dental Research, the National Institute for Allergy and Infectious Diseases, the National Cancer Institute, and the National Institute of Arthritis, Metabolism and Digestive Diseases, all have educational material about nutrition as it applies to their areas of interest. Information can be obtained by contacting them directly or writing to Dr. Artemis Simopoulos, Chairman, Nutrition Coordinating Committee, National Institutes of Health, Bethesda, MD 20205.

• State health departments and some local health departments can be excellent sources of information about nutrition.

Scientific and Professional Organizations

• The American Institute of Nutrition and the American Society for Clinical Nutrition, both mentioned above, are located at 9650 Rockville Pike, Bethesda, MD 20014. ASCN publishes the *American Journal of Clinical Nutrition,* the most widely respected clinical nutrition journal.

• The AMA Department of Foods and Nutrition has pamphlets available and can answer questions. Its address is 535 N. Dearborn St., Chicago, IL 60610. State medical societies may also be helpful.

• The American Dietetic Association has a variety of publications and can answer questions. Its address is 430 N. Michigan Ave., Chicago, IL 60611. State and local dietetic associations are usually eager to be helpful. Dial-A-Dietitian services are available in a number of cities.

• The American Dental Association's Office of Public Information can answer questions about nutrition that pertain to dental health. Its address is 211 E. Chicago Ave., Chicago, IL 60611.

• The National Nutrition Consortium, which issues reports from time to time, may also answer questions. Its address is 2121 P St., Washington, DC 20037.

• The Institute of Food Technologists issues scientific summaries and position papers on topics related to food processing. Its address is 221 N. LaSalle St., Chicago, IL 60601. IFT also has communicators available for media interviews in more than 30 cities.

• The Nutrition Foundation publishes reports and the journal, *Nutrition Reviews.* The address of its office of education is 887 17th Street, N.W., Washington, DC 20006.

• The Society for Nutrition Education publishes the *Journal of Nutrition Education* and a variety of other educational materials. Its address is 1736 Franklin Street, Oakland, CA 94612.

• Accredited colleges and medical schools with nutrition departments may be excellent sources of information.

Voluntary Agencies

Many voluntary agencies provide information about nutrition as it applies to their areas of special interest. Most notable are:

- American Cancer Society, 777 3rd Ave., New York, NY 10017
- American Diabetes Association, 600 5th Avenue, New York, NY 10020
- American Heart Association, 7370 Greenville Ave., Dallas, TX 75231
- Arthritis Foundation, 3400 Peachtree Rd., Atlanta, GA 30326
- Asthma and Allergy Foundation of America, 801 2nd Ave., New York, NY 10017
- Juvenile Diabetes Foundation, 23 E. 26th St., New York, NY 10023

Consumer Protection Organizations

- The American Council on Science and Health has a special interest in chemical and nutritional issues in our lives. Membership, open to anyone, costs $35/year. Several times a year, ACSH publishes reports based upon thorough review of current scientific evidence on particular topics. It also publishes a bimonthly newsletter and maintains a speakers bureau. Its address is 1995 Broadway, New York, NY 10023.
- Better Business Bureaus located in many cities can sometimes provide information about products sold with nutrition or health claims. The National Advertising Division of the Council of Better Business Bureaus, Inc., can often exert considerable pressure on companies which cannot justify questionable claims made in national advertising. Its address is 845 3rd Ave., New York, NY 10022.
- The California Council Against Health Fraud, Inc., investigates questionable methods, publishes a monthly newsletter about political developments in the area of quackery, and maintains a speakers bureau. Information about membership, which costs $10/year, can be obtained by writing to William T. Jarvis, Ph.D., P.O. Box 1276, Loma Linda, CA 92354.
- The Lehigh Valley Committee Against Health Fraud, Inc., P.O. Box 1602, Allentown, PA 18105, maintains a clearinghouse for information about quackery, health frauds and consumer health. Its major publication, *The Health Robbers,* has achieved widespread acclaim and is already in its second edition. A few years ago, the Committee received the following letter:

Gentlemen: I've just finished reading "The Health Robbers" and found it to be quite an eye-opener. I've been interested in nutrition for the past three years or so, spurred on by chronic fatigue and encouraging friends. Naturally, I've been ingesting food supplements by the handfuls, reading *Prevention* and related books, worrying about "harmful" things in my family's diet, and getting all kinds of static from my kids. Recently I determined to try to find out what is the right course to pursue, nutritionally, for my family and me, and yours was the first book I came across in the library relative to my search. I believe what it says and have experienced a definite sense of release after reading it. Yesterday I put all my vitamin bottles away and I don't mind telling you it was scary! (Is this whole movement based on fear?)

It certainly is. The great American hustle, with its deceptions and temptations, is deeply ingrained in our society. But if you have the courage to live in the real world, this book can help you find it.

A Final Comment

This book was written to protect you from being a victim of the great American hustle. We hope it will also arouse you to take action.

We need your help. If you have been helped by this book, please do the following:

1. Recommend the book to your friends.
2. Urge your local school and public libraries to obtain copies.
3. Ask the editors of publications to which you subscribe to review the book.
4. Report questionable health matters to appropriate federal agencies and to us. Complaints about mail-order frauds should be sent to the Postal Service. Complaints about product labeling should be sent to the FDA. Complaints about other advertising should be sent to both the FDA and the Federal Trade Commission. Complaints about national advertising should also be sent to the National Advertising Division of the Council of Better Business Bureaus. Addresses of these agencies are listed in Chapter 13.

Remember, in matters of health there should be no tolerance for deception. Your effort in opposing quackery may save many people from being hurt—and may even save a life!

—The Lehigh Valley Committee
Against Health Fraud, Inc.
P.O. Box 1602
Allentown, PA 18105
215-437-1795

166

Toxic Reactions to Plant Products Sold in Health Food Stores

Some of the plant materials sold in health food stores, particularly herbal teas, may be harmful. Such teas, may have only a single ingredient or may be blends of as many as 20 different kinds of leaves, seeds and flowers.

Two teas with diuretic action should be avoided because of their toxic effects. *Juniper* berries can irritate the gastrointestinal tract. *Shave grass* or *horsetail* plants contain nicotine and thiaminase; in horses and other grazing animals, these plants have caused excitement, loss of appetite and muscular control, diarrhea, labored breathing, convulsions, coma and death. Thiamine deficiency with classical signs of beriberi has been reported in sheep after experimental administration of shave grass.

Herbal teas containing *buckthorn* bark and *senna* leaves, flowers and bark have caused severe diarrhea. *Dock* roots and *aloe* leaves are also powerful laxatives available as teas. Aloe is a particularly strong laxative widely used in veterinary medicine for constipated large animals.

Ingestion of half a cup of *burdock root* tea purchased in a health food store has resulted in typical anticholinergic symptoms of blurred vision with enlarged pupils, dry mouth, inability to urinate, and bizarre behavior and speech, including hallucinations. High levels of an atropine-like alkaloid were found in the tea and may have represented an unidentified contaminant. A number of other herbs that are either smoked or used in tea contain anticholinergics and other substances that may have euphoric, stimulant or hallucinogenic effects. These include such common plants as *catnip, juniper, hydrangea, lobelia, jimson weed* and *wormwood. Nutmeg* can cause hallucinations, and very high doses can cause liver damage and death. It is not commonly abused, however, because even fairly small amounts can cause severe headaches, cramps and nausea.

Camomile (*chamomile*) tea is available in health food stores under many brand names. Tea made from its flower heads may cause skin reactions, anaphylactic shock, and other severe hypersensitivity reactions in people allergic to ragweed, asters, chrysanthemums or other members of the Compositae family. Patients allergic to any member of this family should also avoid teas made from floral heads of *goldenrod, marigold* and *yarrow*. Delayed hypersensitivity has occurred after drinking tea made from the leaves of *St. John's Wort.*

Licorice root in large amounts can cause sodium and water retention, low blood potassium, high blood pressure, heart failure and stoppage of the heart.

Devil's claw root, which was recently introduced from South Africa as a tea, can make the uterus contract and should be avoided during pregnancy. *Pennyroyal* oil has caused death due to kidney and liver poisoning.

Sassafras root bark contains sassafras oil that is at least 70 percent safrole, a substance that is toxic to the liver and can cause cancer in animals.

Ginseng contains small amounts of estrogens and has been reported to cause swollen and painful breasts. Other substances may also be packaged and sold as ginseng, including *mandrake* root, which contains scopolamine (a hallucinogen) and *reserpine* (which can lower blood pressure).

Indian tobacco, which is smoked or used in tea, contains lobeline, a central nervous system stimulant similar to nicotine. Ingestion in large doses can cause sweating, vomiting, paralysis, depressed temperature, coma and death.

Mistletoe leaves, stems and berries contain toxic amines and proteins that may cause gastroenteritis. Some toxins in mistletoe produce the same effects in experimental animals as the injection of a heart toxin from cobra venom.

The entire *poke* plant (pokeweed, inkberry), and particularly the root, is toxic. Eating the uncooked plant can cause gastroenteritis, decreased breathing, and death. Children have died from eating the berries. Pokeweed also contains a "mitogen," a substance which may cause cells to multiply in harmful ways.

Seeds or pits, bark and leaves of *apricot, bitter almond, certain beans, cherry, choke cherry, peach, pear, apple* and *plum* contain compounds, which, after being eaten, liberate hydrogen cyanide, sometimes in sufficient quantities to cause cyanide poisoning. Children have been poisoned and some have died after eating such seeds. Adults have also been poisoned by drinking milkshakes that included apricot kernels. Goiter, staggering gait, nerve damage and blindness have all been linked to chronic cyanide poisoning caused by eating *cassava.*

The ingredients of some teas may be labeled incorrectly, and errors can occur in identification of herbs by suppliers; severe liver damage from pyrrolizidine alkaloids has been documented because of such an error. In another report, pyrrolizidine alkaloids apparently contained in *mate* tea caused liver damage and death in a woman who drank large amount of the tea for a period of years.

The above information has been adapted, with the kind permission of its editor, from the April 6, 1979 issue of *The Medical Letter.* Many other types of toxic plant products are described in the book, *Toxicants Occurring Naturally in Foods,* published in 1973 by the National Academy of Sciences.

Appendix B

Daily Food Guide

This Guide, developed by the United States Department of Agriculture and modified by us, tells you the kinds and amounts of foods that make up a nutritious diet. But it lets *you* make the choices to fit your eating style and needs.

The Guide divides commonly eaten foods into five groups according to the nutritional contributions they make. By following it, you'll be choosing foods adequate in vitamins, minerals and protein, as well as appropriate in calorie content.

Calories are a measure of the energy which food provides. The extra calories that you get and your body does not use up are stored as fat. The suggested number of servings in the Guide average about 1,200 calories, provide adequate protein, and supply the vitamins and minerals you need daily. Planning your day's food around this foundation will automatically give you a balanced diet.

Making the Guide Work for You

You can personalize the Guide by fitting it to your calorie needs. All foods, except water and noncaloric drinks, have calories. Nutritionally, there are no "good calories" or "bad calories." Some foods give you little *but* calories, while others give you calories *plus* nutrients.

How many calories you need depends upon how much energy you use up. Generally, older people need fewer calories than younger people, women need fewer than men, and bridge players and bookkeepers need fewer than tennis players and construction workers.

If you are gaining unwanted weight, or if you want to lose weight, cut down first from the fifth group (fats-sweets-alcohol). If you are still gaining weight, cut down next on portion sizes from the other groups. Cut *down*, but don't cut *out*, and select the lower calorie foods within each group. On the other hand, if you want to gain weight, eat larger or additional portions from the first four groups and include more foods from the fifth group.

170

Remember, this Guide gives you only the basics. You have to choose foods which meet your special needs and tastes. But it is usually best to eat a wide assortment of foods from the first four groups (the "Basic Four").

VEGETABLE AND FRUIT GROUP

Four Basic Servings Daily
Include one good vitamin C source such as a citrus fruit or juice each day. Also frequently include deep yellow or dark green vegetables (for vitamin A) and unpeeled fruits and vegetables and those with edible seeds, such as berries (for fiber).

What's a Serving?

For all fruits and vegetables count either ½ cup or a typical portion. Examples: one orange, half a medium grapefruit or cantaloupe, juice of one lemon, a wedge of lettuce, a bowl of salad, or one medium potato.

What's in it for You?

This group is important for its contribution of vitamins A, C, B_1 (thiamine) and B_6 (pyridoxine) and fiber, although individual foods in this group vary widely in how much of these they provide. That's why a wide variety should be eaten. Dark green and deep yellow vegetables are good sources of vitamin A. Most dark green vegetables, if not overcooked, are also reliable sources of vitamin C and folic acid (folacin)—as are citrus fruits (oranges, grapefruits, tangerines, lemons), melons, berries and tomatoes. Dark green vegetables are valued for riboflavin (vitamin B_2), folacin, iron and magnesium as well. Certain greens—collards, kale, mustard, turnip and dandelion—provide calcium. Nearly all vegetables and fruits are low in fat, and none contains cholesterol.

BREAD AND CEREAL GROUP

Four Basic Servings Daily
Select whole-grain and enriched or fortified products.

What's a Serving?

This group includes all products made with whole grains or enriched flour or meal, including bread, biscuits, muffins, waffles, pancakes, cooked or ready-to-eat cereals, cornmeal, flour, grits, macaroni and spaghetti, noodles, rice, rolled oats, barley and bulgur.

Count as a serving 1 slice of bread, 1 ounce of ready-to-eat cereal, or ½ to ¾ cup of cooked cereal, cornmeal, grits, macaroni, noodles, rice or spaghetti.

What's in it for You?

These whole-grain or enriched foods are important sources of B vitamins. They also provide protein and are a major source of this nutrient in vegetarian diets. Whole-grain products contain more fiber.

Most breakfast cereals are enriched at nutrient levels higher than those occurring in natural whole grain. In fact, some fortification adds vitamins not normally found in cereals (vitamins A, B_{12}, C and D). These extra vitamins are unnecessary if you are eating a balanced diet. There is no nutritional reason to pay inflated prices for over-fortified breakfast cereals to obtain vitamins present in other foods in your diet.

MILK AND CHEESE GROUP

Basic Servings Daily

Children under 9	2 to 3 servings	Adults	2 servings
Children 9 to 12	3 servings	Pregnant Women	3 servings
Teens	4 servings	Nursing Mothers	4 servings

What's a Serving?

This group includes milk in any form: whole, skim, lowfat, evaporated, buttermilk and nonfat dry milk. Also yogurt, ice cream, ice milk and cheese, including cottage cheese. Count one 8-ounce cup of milk as a serving. Common portions of some dairy products and their milk equivalents in calcium are:

1 cup plain yogurt	= 1 cup milk
1 ounce Cheddar or Swiss cheese (natural or process)	= ¾ cup milk
1- inch cube Cheddar or Swiss cheese	= ½ cup milk
1 ounce process cheese food	= ½ cup milk
½ cup ice cream or ice milk	= ⅓ cup milk
1 tablespoon or ½ ounce process cheese spread; or 1 tablespoon Parmesan cheese	= ¼ cup milk
½ cup cottage cheese	= ¼ cup milk

Note: You'll get about the same amount of calcium in each of these portions, but varying amounts of calories.

Milk used in cooked foods—such as creamed soups, sauces and puddings—can count toward filling your daily quota in this group.

What's in it for You?

Milk and most milk products are the major source of calcium in the American diet. They contribute riboflavin, protein and vitamins A, B_6, and B_{12}, and also provide vitamin D when fortified with this vitamin. Fortified (with vitamins A and D) lowfat or skim milk products have most of the nutrients of whole milk products, but have fewer calories.

MEAT, POULTRY, FISH AND BEANS GROUP
Two Basic Servings Daily

What's a Serving?

This group includes beef, veal, lamb, pork, poultry, fish, shellfish (shrimp, oysters, crabs, etc.), organ meats (liver, kidneys, etc.), dry beans or peas, soybeans, lentils, eggs, seeds, nuts, peanuts and peanut butter. Count 2 to 3 ounces of lean, cooked meat, poultry or fish without bone as a serving. One egg, ½ to ¾ cup of cooked dry beans, dry peas, soybeans or lentils, 2 tablespoons of peanut butter, and ¼ to ½ cup of nuts, sesame seeds or sunflower seeds count as 1 ounce of meat, poultry or fish.

What's in it for You?

These foods are valued for the protein, phosphorus, vitamins B_6, B_{12} and other vitamins and minerals they provide. However, only foods of animal origin contain B_{12} naturally. It's a good idea to vary your choices among these foods as each has distinct nutritional advantages. For example, red meats and oysters are good sources of zinc. Liver and egg yolks are valuable sources of vitamin A. Dry beans, dry peas, soybeans and nuts are worthwhile sources of magnesium. The flesh of fish and poultry is relatively low in calories and saturated fat. Seeds (such as sunflower or sesame) contribute polyunsaturated fatty acids.

Cholesterol, like vitamin B_{12}, occurs naturally only in foods of animal origin. We get about 15 percent of our cholesterol from our food and synthesize the rest in our livers and other body cells. All meats contain cholesterol, which is present in both the lean and the fat. The highest concentration is found in brain, other organ meats, and egg yolks. Fish and shellfish, except for shrimp, are relatively low in cholesterol. Dairy products also supply dietary cholesterol, but contain other substances which lower blood cholesterol by reducing cholesterol synthesis.

Is getting enough iron a problem? It can be, particularly for young children, teenage girls and menstruating women. Meats are reliable sources of iron absorbable by the body. Whole-grain and enriched breads and cereals, dry beans and dry peas, and various other vegetables also contain iron. But the iron in these foods is well absorbed only when they are eaten at the same time as a good source of vitamin C (such as orange juice) or along with meat. Tea and coffee inhibit iron absorption from plant products, but not from meat.

FATS, SWEETS AND ALCOHOL GROUP

In general, the amount of these foods to use depends on the number of calories you require. It's a good idea to concentrate first on the nutrient-rich foods provided in the other four groups as the basis of your daily diet.

What's a Serving?

This group includes foods like butter, margarine, mayonnaise and other salad dressings, and other fats and oils; candy, sugar, jams, jellies, syrup, sweet toppings and other sweets; soft drinks and other highly sugared beverages; and alcoholic beverages such as wine, beer and liquor. Also included are refined but unenriched breads, pastries and flour products. Some of these foods are used as ingredients in prepared foods or are added to other foods at the table. Others are just "extras." No serving sizes are defined because a basic number of servings is not suggested for this group.

What's in it for You?

These products, with some exceptions such as vegetable oils, provide mainly calories. Vegetable oils generally supply vitamin E and essential fatty acids. Carbohydrates (starches or sugars) and proteins have 4 calories per gram. Fats and oils have 9 calories per gram, but keep hunger pangs away longer. Alcohol has 7 calories per gram, but few alcoholic beverages are 100 percent alcohol. Generally, the higher the alcoholic content, the higher the calories per gram.

Unenriched, refined bakery products are included here because, like other foods and beverages in this group, they usually provide relatively low levels of vitamins, minerals and protein compared with calories.

Appendix C

Recommended Reading

Anti-Quackery Books

The Health Robbers, 2nd edition, edited by Stephen Barrett, M.D. 1980. A comprehensive expose of quackery. $12.95. George F. Stickley Co., 210 West Washington Square, Philadelphia, PA 19106.

Health Quackery, by Consumers Union. 1980. Excellent discussions of chiropractic, hypoglycemia, laetrile, arthritis and weight-reduction quackery, vitamin E, antifluoridation propaganda, mail-order frauds and other selected topics. $5.00. Consumer Reports Books, Orangeburg, NY 10962.

The Medical Messiahs, by James Harvey Young, Ph.D. 1967. A history of the government's struggle against patent medicines in the 20th Century. $5.95. Princeton University Press.

The New Nuts Among the Berries, by Ronald Deutsch. 1977. Factual but amusing account of how nutrition nonsense captured America. $5.95. Bull Publishing Co., P.O. Box 208, Palo Alto, CA 94302.

The Tooth Robbers, edited by Stephen Barrett, M.D., and Sheldon Rovin, D.D.S. 1980. A pro-fluoridation handbook for community leaders and other interested citizens. $8.50. George F. Stickley Co., Phila.

Nutrition Cultism, by Victor Herbert, M.D., J.D. 1980. Detailed discussion of laetrile, "B_{15}," vitamin facts and fallacies, dangers of megavitamins. $12.95. George F. Stickley Co., Phila.

Nutrition Misinformation and Food Faddism, 1974. A collection of 17 excellent papers. $2.50. The Nutrition Foundation, 888 17th St., N.W., Washington, DC 20006.

Megavitamin and Orthomolecular Therapy in Psychiatry, 1973 An American Psychiatric Association Task Force Report. $3.00. APA Publications Services, 1700 N. 18th St., N.W., Washington, DC 20009

The Vitamin Conspiracy, by John Fried. 1975. A brilliant analysis of the megavitamin "controversy." Out-of-print. E. P. Dutton Co., 2 Park Avenue, New York, NY 10016.

175

At Your Own Risk—The Case Against Chiropractic, by Ralph Lee Smith. 1969. Simon and Schuster. This book is out-of-print, but not out of date. It is available for $3.00 from LVCAHF, Inc., P.O. Box 1602, Allentown, PA 18105.

A Study of Health Practices and Opinions, 1972. FDA survey of health and nutrition attitudes of a large number of individuals. $26.00. Order publication #PB-210978 from the National Technical Information Service, 5285 Port Royal Road, Springfield, VA 22161.

General Nutrition

Realities of Nutrition, by Ronald Deutsch. 1976. Easy-to-read discussion of the fallacies and realities of nutrients. $9.95. Bull Publishing Co.

Nautilus Nutrition Book, by Ellington Darden, Ph.D. 1981. Easy-to-read questions and answers about basic nutrition. $7.95. Contemporary Books.

Food, by the United States Department of Agriculture. 1979. Covers food choices, dietary principles, menu guides and recipes. $3.25. Order publication #G-228 from the Supt. of Documents, U.S. Govt. Printing Office, Washington, DC 20402.

The No-Nonsense Guide to Food and Nutrition, by Marion McGill and Orrea Pye. 1978. An easy-to-read reference book. $5.95. Butterick Publishing, 708 3rd Ave., New York, NY 10017.

Eat OK-Feel-OK—Food Facts and Your Health, by Fredrick J. Stare, M.D., and Elizabeth M. Whelan, Sc.D. 1978. Basic nutritional concepts plus rebuttal of misinformation. $9.75 Christopher Publishing House, 53 Billings Rd., North Quincy, MA 02171.

Special Topics

Nutrition References and Book Reviews 1981. A reliable guide to nutrition books. Especially useful to librarians and educators. $8.00. Chicago Nutrition Association, 8158 S. Kedsie Ave., Chicago, IL 60652.

Recommended Dietary Allowances, 9th Edition, 1980. A detailed scientific discussion of nutrient needs. $6.00. National Academy of Sciences, 2101 Constitution Ave., Washington, DC 20418.

A Guide to Good Nutrition during and after Chemotherapy and Radiation, by S. Aker and P. Lenssen. 1979. Solutions to eating problems of cancer patients undergoing intensive treatment. Send

$3.50 to Dietary Services, Fred Hutchinson Cancer Research Center, 1124 Columbia St., Seattle, WA 98014.

Vitamin Safety, published by the National Nutrition Consortium. Available for $2.50 from the American Dietetic Association, 430 N. Michigan Ave., Chicago, IL 60611.

Nutrition and Athletic Performance, by Ellington Darden, Ph.D. 1976. Basic information from a nutrition expert who is also a former athlete. $3.95. The Athletic Press, P.O. Box 23 L4-D, Pasadena, CA 91105.

Food for Sport, by Nathan Smith, M.D. 1975. A basic guide for athletes. $5.95. Bull Publishing Co.

Food Allergy, by Frederic Speer. 1978. A practical approach to the management of food allergies, with major emphasis on identification of problem foods. $16.00. Publishing Sciences Group, Inc., 411 Massachusetts Ave., Acton, MA 01720.

The Pain of Obesity, by Albert J. Stunkard, M.D. 1976. Case histories and discussion of treatment written for a lay audience. $9.75. Bull Publishing Co.

Change Your Habits to Change Your Shape—For Teenagers Only, by J. Ideka. 1978. Practical information on weight control. $5.95. Bull Publishing Co.

The Vegetarian Handbook: A Guide to Vegetarian Nutrition, by Roger Doyle. 1979. A good source of information for someone who chooses to become a vegetarian. $6.95. Crown Publishers, 1 Park Avenue, New York, NY 10016.

The Parent's Guide to Weight Control for Children Ages 5 to 13 Years, by B.K. Feig. 1980. Practical guide for weight control of moderately overweight children. $6.95. Charles C Thomas, 301-27 E. Lawrence Ave., Springfield, IL 62717.

Cookbooks   •

The American Heart Association Cookbook, edited by Ruthe Eshleman and Mary Winston. 1979. Contains more than 550 recipes for people concerned about their caloric, fat and cholesterol intake. $12.95. David McKay Co., Inc., 2 Park Ave., New York, NY 10016.

Cooking Without Your Salt Shaker, produced by the Northeast Ohio Affiliate of the American Heart Association. 1978. More than 150 recipes for low-salt, modified fat diets. $5.00 (Order through your local Heart Association.)

The Family Cookbook, compiled by the American Diabetes Association and the American Dietetic Association. 1980. Principles of dietary management of diabetes, plus more than 250 recipes. $12.95. Prentice-Hall, Inc., Englewood Cliffs, NJ 07632.

Textbooks

Modern Nutrition in Health and Disease, 6th edition, edited by Robert S. Goodhart, M.D., D.M.S., and Maurice E. Shils, M.D., Sc.D. 1980. A comprehensive text and reference book for students and professionals. $47.50. Lea & Febiger, 600 Washington Square, Philadelphia, PA 19106.

Nutrition and Drug Interrelations, edited by John N. Hathcock and Julius Coon. 1978. $58.00. Academic Press, Inc., 111 5th Ave., New York, NY 10003.

Geriatric Nutrition, by Annette B. Natow et al. 1980. Provides nutrition information for health professionals who work with older adults. $15.95. CBI Publishing Co., Inc., 51 Sleeper St., Boston, MA 02210.

Foundations of Food Preparation, by Gladys C. Peckham and Jeanne H. Freeland-Graves. 1979. A text aimed at first-level college students majoring in food and nutrition. $15.95. Macmillan Publishing Co., Inc., 866 3rd Ave., New York, NY 10022.

Nutrition and Diet Therapy, by S. Williams. 1977. A basic textbook. $17.95. C. V. Mosby Co., 11830 Westline Industrial Drive, St. Louis, MO 63141.

The Science of Food, by Marion Bennion. 1980. An advanced textbook. $19.50. Harper & Row, 10 E. 53rd St., New York, NY 10022.

Food: The Gift of Osiris, by William J. Darby et al. 1977. A scholarly account of food use in ancient times and the effect of ancient beliefs upon modern food usage. $83 for 2-volume set. Academic Press.

Contemporary Nutrition Controversies, edited by Theodore P. Labuza, Ph.D., and A. Elizabeth Sloan, Ph.D. 1979. Discussion of issues perceived as important by the general public. Designed primarily for use in college classes for non-majors in nutrition. $11.95. West Publishing Co., 50 W. Kellogg Blvd., St. Paul, MN 55165.

Magazines

Consumer Reports. Excellent monthly magazine which tests products and also reports on a wide variety of consumer issues. Health and nutrition topics are frequently covered. $12/yr. Consumer Reports, Orangeburg, NY 10962.

FDA Consumer. Excellent monthly magazine which includes frequent articles about health, nutrition and food safety. $12/yr. from Consumer Information, Pueblo, CO 81009.

Nutrition Today. $14.75/yr. Issued bimonthly by the Nutrition Today Society, P.O. Box 1829, Annapolis, MD 21404.

Newsletters

Contemporary Nutrition. Issued monthly, free-of-charge to health and nutrition professionals and other selected individuals. Back issues are $4.00 per set. Requests should be mailed to G. T. Florey, Assistant Editor, General Mills, P.O. Box 1112, Dept. 65, Minneapolis, MN 55440.

Nutrition News. Issued quarterly, free-of-charge to health and nutrition professionals, by the National Dairy Council, 6300 N. River Rd., Rosemont, IL 60061.

Dairy Council Digest. Scientific summaries issued bimonthly by the National Dairy Council. Free-of-charge to health and nutrition professionals.

The Medical Letter. Biweekly report on drugs and therapeutics (including questionable "nutrition" remedies). Although written primarily for physicians, it is also useful to medical journalists. $22.50/yr.; or $11.25 for physicians in training. 56 Harrison Street, New Rochelle, NY 10801.

Pamphlets

The Healthy Approach to Slimming, 1978. A 21-page booklet prepared by the American Medical Association. Send $1.00 for pamphlet #OP-003 to AMA Order Dept., P.O. Box 821, Monroe, WI 53566.

Fluoridation Facts—Answers to Questions About Fluoridation, 1981. A 36-page booklet available from the American Dental Association. Single copies free, $10.25 for 25 copies, $38.95 for 100 copies from ADA Order Dept., 211 East Chicago Ave., Chicago, IL 60611.

Eating Hints—Recipes and Tips for Better Nutrition During Cancer Treatment. An 86-page booklet available free-of-charge from the National Cancer Institute, Bethesda, MD 20205.

Index

181

International Academy of Preventive Medicine (IAPM), 69, 106
International Association of Cancer Victims and Friends (IACVF), 112
International College of Applied Nutrition, 69
International Health Institute (IHI), 58-59
International Society for Fluoride Research, 106
Iridology (iridiagnosis), 65
Iron, deficiency in vegetarians, 8, need for, 8, sources of, 51, 174, toxicity of, 51
Iron-deficiency anemia, management of, 51
Irons, Victor Earl, 118
Jacobson, Michael, 105
Jarvis, D. C., 89
Jarvis, William, 128
Jensen, Bernard, 65, 123
J. I. Rodale, Ltd., 100-101
John Beard Memorial Foundation, 110
John Birch Society, 113
Journalism, peer review in, 144-147
J. B. Williams Co., 50-51, 151
Jukes, Thomas H., 83
Juniper berries, toxic effects of, 167
Kefauver-Harris Amendment to Food, Drug and Cosmetic Act, 93, 149
Kelley, William D., 58-59
Kellogg, John Harvey, 87
Kellogg Company, development of, 87-88
Kinesiology, 68
Knight, Gilda, 106
Koch, William, 19
Kordel, Lelord, 90
Krebs, Byron, 110
Krebs, Ernst T., Jr., 20, 110-111
Krebs, Ernst T., Sr., 20, 109-110
Labeling, FDA definition of, 149, laws, enforcement of, by FDA, 158
Labels, therapeutic claims on, 32-33
Laetrile, 20, 71, 108-115, court cases concerning, 110, 113-114, 121-122, 134-135, 152, drive to legalize, 113-115, effectiveness, lack of, 108, 109, shifting claims for, 109, individuals promoting, 109-112, National Cancer Institute test of, 109, NHF promotion of, 133-135, other organizations promoting, 112-113, supporters, arguments of, 114

Laetrile Case Histories (Richardson and Griffin), 111-112
Laetrile: Control of Cancer (Kittler), 112
LaForte, Dom, 126
Larchmont Books, 35
Larsen, Glenn Harold, 128
Law(s), effectiveness of, 152-155, FDA, 148-150, FTC, 150-151, postal, 148, weakness of, 148-158
Law Enforcement Report, 150
Lecturers, prominent, selling power of, 36
Lee, Royal S., 60-61, 116-117
Lee, William H., 49
Lee Foundation for Nutritional Research, 117
Lefkowitz, Louis, hearing on organic foods, 73, 75
Lehigh Valley Committee Against Health Fraud, 70, 71, 101-102, 124, 129, 134, 137, 140, 152, 154, 157, 164, 166
Let's Eat Right to Keep Fit (Davis), 94
Let's Get Well (Davis), 94-95
Let's Have Healthy Children (Davis), 157
Let's Live magazine, and hair analysis, 45
Libel, threat of, fighting of misinformation and, 142-144.
Licorice root, toxic effects of, 168
Lifelines, 43
Linblads, Inc., 61-62, 154
Linn, Robert, 107
Linus Pauling Institute of Medicine, The, 96
Look Younger, Live Longer (Hauser), 89
Low blood sugar. See "Hypoglycemia"
Macfadden, Bernarr, 26, 88-89
Magazines, use by retailers to generate sales, 35, recommended, 178-179
Manner, Harold, 62
Manner Metabolic Therapy Program, 62
Manure, as fertilzier, disadvantages of, 12, 76
Mayer, Jean, 105
Mayo Clinic, 114
McDonald, Larry, 114, 134
McNaughton, Andrew R. L., 122
Meat, daily servings of, 173
Media, nutrition and the, 139-147, 152
Medical facts, determination of, 1-3
"Medical Freedom of Choice" bill, 132
Medical knowledge, development of, 1-3

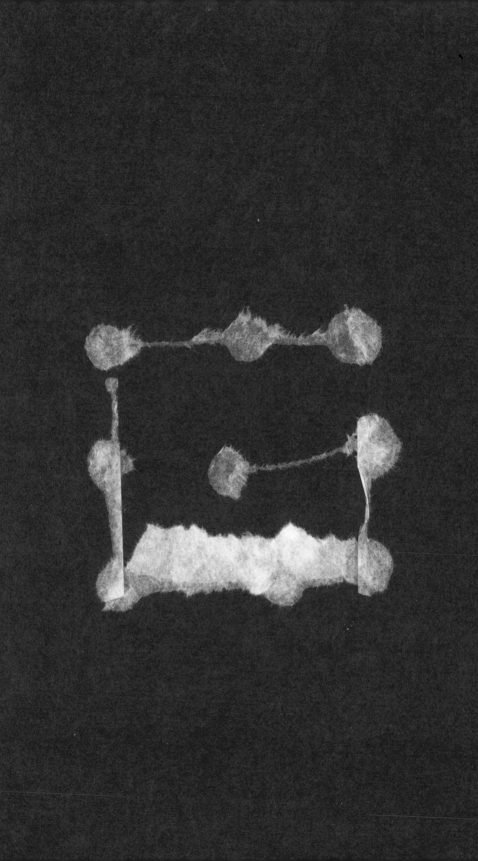